Food for Life

The Cancer Prevention Cookbook

RICHARD BOHANNON, M.D.,
TERRI PISCHOFF AND KATHY PAKOSH

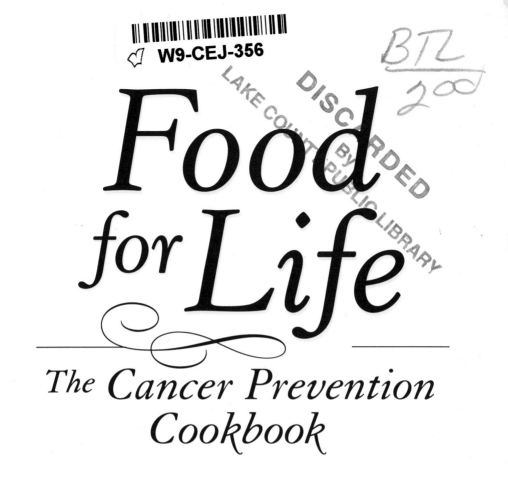

CB
CONTEMPORARY BOOKS

Library of Congress Cataloging-in-Publication Data

Bohannon, Richard.
  Food for Life : the cancer prevention cookbook / Richard Bohannon,
Terri Pischoff, and Kathy M. Pakosh. — Rev. ed.
    p. cm.
  Includes index.
  ISBN 0-8092-2845-9
  1. Cancer—Diet therapy—Recipes. 2. Cancer—Prevention.
3. Cancer—Nutritional aspects. I. Pischoff, Terri. II. Pakosh,
Kathy M. III. Title.
  RC271.D52B64   1998
  616.99'40654—dc21   98-15348
                                                          CIP

Cover design by Monica Baziuk
Cover illustration copyright © Barbara Maslen/Stock Illustration Source
Interior design by Precision Graphics
Interior illustrations by Kent Snodgrass/Precision Graphics

Published by Contemporary Books
A division of NTC/Contemporary Publishing Group, Inc.
4255 West Touhy Avenue, Lincolnwood (Chicago), Illinois 60646-1975 U.S.A.
International Standard Book Number: 0-8092-2845-9

15   14   13   12   11   10   9   8   7   6   5   4   3   2   1

*This book is dedicated
with much love and great admiration
to Dorothy McIntosh
for overcoming her cancer.*

*Dr. Bohannon and Kathy Pakosh have selected
the following charities for their donations:
the American Cancer Society,
the Susan G. Komen Breast Cancer Foundation,
and CaP Cure (Prostate Cancer Foundation).*

CONTENTS

ACKNOWLEDGMENTS

We thank the many people who helped us with our project. Special thanks to Dr. Nancy Bohannon, M.D., endocrinologist; to Dr. Mark Messina, M.D., for his lengthy interview highlighting his research on nutrition and its relationship to disease prevention; to Maureen Pakosh, medical librarian, for her expertise; to Marge Harris, our computer expert and general adviser; to Colleen Colman, our typist, who spent many nights and weekends perfecting the manuscript; and to Susan Schwartz, our editor, for her insight, guidance, and patience. Last, but certainly most important, Dr. Bohannon's patients, battling cancer, for their courage and faith.

Each of us would like to add a personal note:

Richard Bohannon: I thank my wife and partner in life, Nancy, and our son, Robert, for their love and support.

Kathy Pakosh: Thank you to my beloved husband, Donald, and my two sons, Daniel and Peter (my greatest accomplishments), for their enthusiasm and encouragement.

Terri Pischoff: Thank you to my dad for teaching me everything he knows about cooking, and to my mother, daughters, and siblings just for being themselves. Thanks also to three mentors: Michael Castleman, Martha Casselman, and Julia Child—all of whom encouraged me to pursue my career as a food writer.

INTRODUCTION

Thirty-five percent of cancer deaths are attributable to diet alone.

Researchers at the National Cancer Institute, 1996

Despite the fact that reducing the risk of cancer through diet has been studied for more than 50 years, only in the last 10 years has the subject been widely publicized. When we first published *Food for Life* in 1986, using the American Cancer Society's guidelines for a cancer risk-reduction diet, some of my colleagues in the medical community gave little credence to the idea that what we eat might influence our chances of developing cancer.

Most of them have since conceded that cancer prevention through diet is not only essential, but also vital to the treatment of their patients in general. Beginning at the age of two years (children under the age of two have special dietary needs), everybody needs to be aware of cancer prevention through dietary modification. The estimates from myriad researchers worldwide are firm that 30 to 40 percent of all cancers are related to dietary factors alone. The best cancer prevention tool is the food we put into our mouths.

The impact of these percentages is riveting—we *do* have control over cancer, starting in our own kitchens and using our personal knowledge bank.

As the millennium approaches, we as individuals will be taking even greater responsibility for our own health care. Managed health care is a reality. Morning news shows and other mass media continually apprise us of the latest scientific findings, current self-help remedies, and newest diagnostic procedures. Nutritional news is consistently one of the most popular topics in both print and electronic formats. Virtually unknown by the public 20 years ago, science and medicine as they relate to disease prevention through good nutrition have been demystified. You can't turn on a morning news program without hearing about food and health. Terms such as HDL and LDL levels of cholesterol, antioxidants, free radicals, percentage of calories from fat, soluble and insoluble fiber, and monounsaturated and polyunsaturated fats are familiar today. The old adage "You are what you eat" has never been truer or more important.

While the idea of cancer-preventive nutrition is now widely accepted, most people are too busy with life to think daily of dietary benefits.

To keep this presentation simple, this section states the basic principles of reducing cancer risk through diet. The individual chapter introductions offer more details about anticancer cooking, food selection, and preparation.

- Restrict fat intake to *no more* than 30 percent of calories from fat.
- Consume 35 grams of dietary fiber each day.
- Eat a variety of fruits and vegetables, especially those high in vitamin C and beta-carotene (studies have shown that the protective effects of beta-carotene and vitamin C in humans are from dietary sources, not vitamin supplements). The American Cancer Society suggests a total of five portions of fruits and vegetables a day.
- If you drink alcohol, do so only in moderation.
- Limit consumption of foods containing nitrites and nitrates (such as bacon and packaged cold cuts).
- Limit consumption of smoked or barbecued foods to no more than once a week.
- Maintain a healthy weight (eating too many calories, whether from fat, protein, or carbohydrates, increases your chance of contracting many types of cancer).
- Be physically active—do some kind of moderate activity for 30 minutes or more, three times a week.

What about cholesterol? You will notice that in this new edition we include cholesterol in our nutritional analysis. Is there a direct causal relationship between high serum cholesterol levels and cancer? The answer is no. However, a high serum cholesterol level is always a red flag signaling the possibility of serious health issues. High cholesterol levels are often the result of an abundance of dietary fat, usually resulting in excess body weight. Obesity has been linked to cancers of the prostate, colon, and breast, among other types. A lifelong pattern of eating high-fat foods induces high serum cholesterol and can be a potential risk of developing certain cancers or heart disease. We use the American Heart Association's guideline of 300 milligrams (mg) of cholesterol per day. In this new edition of *Food for Life: The Cancer Prevention Cookbook,* we demonstrate that our recipes are low in both fat and cholesterol.

There has also been much recent and exciting information published about soy and its benefits. For the last decade, American researchers have been studying the effects of soy products and disease prevention. Volumes have been written about the traditional diet of Japanese women and their low incidence of breast cancer; there is evidence, as well as many ongoing studies, suggesting that in addition to low fat consumption and high vegetable intake, soy products play a significant role in protecting these women from contracting breast cancer. There are more than 200 studies in the United States alone being conducted to show the relationship between soy products and cancer prevention. To quote Dr. Mark Messina, former program director of NCI (National Cancer Institute), "According to the latest research, the evidence that soy consumption may reduce the risk of prostate cancer or help delay the growth of existing prostate tumors (although still speculative) is increasingly encouraging." We believe that within the coming decade the consumption of soy products will be strongly recommended in the American diet. We encourage you to include soy products (tofu, miso) in your diet occasionally as a substitute for animal proteins.

If these guidelines sound simple, it is because they are. We aren't suggesting drastic or unattainable diet changes, but rather a redirection of your way of eating and cooking. As we stated in our first edition, you should simply eat more of some foods and *less* of others. We need to eat more fruits, vegetables, whole grains, soy products, legumes, and high-fiber foods. We need to eat less high-fat food, processed meat, and barbecued food.

We all have a hectic schedule, yet there is often nothing more relaxing than making a scrumptious meal for family or friends. Cooking should be pleasurable and relaxing. It can be a great stress reducer. Reducing stress is known to lower the risk for contracting many diseases. In this revised edition, we offer more than 200 varied recipes for every cook. Use our selections for formal dinners, buffet suppers, birthday parties, holiday meals, and most important, family dinners.

We discuss cooking and food preparation in every chapter introduction, as well as giving nutritional analysis of each recipe. (Beta-carotene is presented as i.u., international units of vitamin A.) As you follow our recipes or create your own, you will soon become your family's "designated dietitian."

Use this book to prepare more of the cancer prevention foods listed in the recipes. You will be amazed at how simple yet satisfying a cancer risk-reduction eating plan can be.

Good Health and Bon Appétit!

Appetizers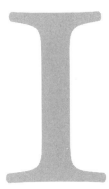

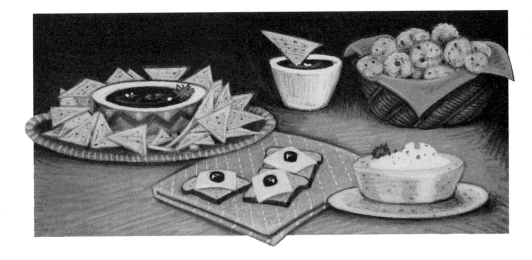

Appetizers are meant to entice and stimulate the palate for the rest of the meal. Because overrich and high-fat concoctions are still too often the typical cocktail party fare, appetizers perhaps are the most difficult recipes to convert to low fat. We have succeeded in keeping all of our appetizers to 30 percent calories from fat or less.

A well-planned array of low-fat appetizers can taste scrumptious, beautify a table, and dazzle your guests with their diverse appeal. A perfect way to begin a party is to gather your friends around a beautifully arranged vegetable platter. Incorporate many foods that are high in either beta-carotene, vitamin C, or both, and are also a good source of dietary fiber—such as carrots, cauliflower, broccoli, turnips, and red and green peppers. These vegetables have a clean, crisp taste, require a minimum of preparation, and are relatively economical. Presented with delicious accompaniments such as Lemon and Chive Dip or Hummus, their eye appeal and taste make them a sure favorite. You can even color coordinate the selection for theme parties.

A few tips will ensure maximum enjoyment of these vegetable trays:

- If you have the time, check local produce stands and farmer's markets for seasonal vegetables. There is a difference in freshness, taste, and usually price—local products being cheaper.

- Do not destroy vitamins by poor storage and handling habits. When you take your vegetables home, rinse them under cool water, pat them dry, and store them in airtight plastic bags or containers in the refrigerator. Some beta-carotene can be lost by wilting or dehydration. Vitamin C is especially susceptible to excess heat and exposure to air, and is soluble in water.

- To make dense vegetables such as broccoli, carrots, turnips, and cauliflower more appealing, you may wish to blanch them (drop them into rapidly boiling water for 3 minutes).

- Don't precut your vegetables hours ahead of time unless you then seal and refrigerate them. Otherwise, they dry out and will look unattractive. Preparing the raw vegetable platter is one of your last tasks before putting the party spread out for your guests.

Many of the appetizers can be made ahead of time without compromising taste or appearance. These include Mushroom Pâté, Hummus, and Warm Vegetable Caviar.

In this chapter we include a number of appetizers that contain cheese as one of the ingredients. Hard cheese has approximately 73 percent calories from fat and, for the most part, should be avoided in quantities more than a sprinkling. However, a number of cheeses are lower in fat and can be used moderately in a cancer risk-reduction diet. These include low-fat or nonfat cottage cheeses, part-skim ricotta, part-skim mozzarella, and part-skim feta. (Always read labels to be sure. The first ingredient should say "part-skim" or "skim milk.") There are other cheeses that are lower in fat than regular cheeses, with advertised names such as low-fat cheddar and Monterey Jack. They can be just as tasty (although higher in sodium) and are usually available at your local supermarket.

Reduced-fat (light) cream cheese also works well in a cancer risk-reduction diet, as shown in Salmon Mousse with Baguettes. We reduce the amount of cream cheese this type of recipe usually demands, substitute a low-fat cream cheese, and add unflavored gelatin to set the mousse. The taste is still rich and creamy with far less fat.

Even using low-fat cheeses, we have kept the amounts to a minimum, using approximately 1 to 2 tablespoons of grated cheese per person for a side dish and approximately ½ cup per person for an entree. We have included cheese in this book because it is a food some people really enjoy (the authors included). We have minimized the fat content without compromising the taste.

For most people, milk products are a major source of calcium. This mineral is necessary for good health and is known to be beneficial in the prevention of osteoporosis. Use skim or low-fat milk products instead of whole milk whenever possible; the amount of calcium per serving remains the same. In some studies, low-fat or skim-milk products along with a vegetable-rich low-fat diet have produced a lower incidence of certain cancers in people who regularly consume them. One cup of yogurt, 2 cups of nonfat cottage cheese, or 1⅓ ounces of natural cheese equal 1 cup of milk.

Appetizers can also be a leisurely first course at a more formal dinner party. Our suggestions would be Lox and Melon with Chives, Mushroom Pâté, Shrimp Dumplings with Sun-Dried Tomato Aioli, and Broccoli Frittata.

This chapter contains a variety of wonderful appetizers with various tastes, textures, and presentations. Wherever feasible, we have minimized the preparation time to 30 minutes or less so you'll have more time to spend with your guests.

Beer Cheese with Rye Toasts

Packed in attractive crocks, this cheese makes a wonderful hostess present or addition to a gift basket.

Makes 12 servings

½ cup beer

12 ounces low-fat cheddar cheese, grated

2 tablespoons flour

2 ounces crumbled blue cheese

2 teaspoons Dijon mustard

1 teaspoon Worcestershire sauce

¼ teaspoon Tabasco

½ cup finely chopped yellow onion

½ cup finely chopped scallion

36 slices of rye melba toast

Open beer and let it stand a few minutes until the foam subsides.

Using a food processor fitted with the steel blade, or an electric mixer, combine the remaining ingredients except the toast. Add the ½ cup beer and mix until creamy. Pack the mixture in crocks, cover them, and refrigerate the cheese for a few days to allow the flavors to develop.

Serve the cheese at room temperature with the rye melba toast.

Nutritional Analysis

Per Serving

Calories (kcal)	152.5	Cholesterol (mg)	10.0
Total Fat (g)	3.8	Dietary Fiber (g)	1.2
Saturated Fat (g)	2.3	% Calories from Fat	28.2
Monounsaturated Fat (g)	1.1	Vitamin C (mg)	3.0
Polyunsaturated Fat (g)	0.3	Vitamin A (i.u.)	117.0

BROCCOLI FRITTATA

A great appetizer, brunch dish, or picnic entree. Broccoli is one of the best vegetables in a cancer risk-reduction eating plan because it is high in beta-carotene, vitamin C, and fiber.

Makes 12 servings

3 tablespoons low-sodium chicken broth

⅔ cup finely chopped yellow onion

⅓ cup finely chopped green bell pepper

3 cloves garlic, minced

1 20-ounce package frozen chopped broccoli, defrosted and drained

1 teaspoon dried oregano

½ teaspoon salt

½ teaspoon black pepper

5 drops Tabasco

⅓ cup finely chopped fresh parsley

4 egg whites

¼ cup grated Asiago cheese

3 tablespoons dry unseasoned bread crumbs

Paprika

Preheat the oven to 350°F. Coat a 9" × 13" pan with cooking spray.

Heat the broth in a skillet over medium heat until it boils. Add the onion, bell pepper, and garlic and sauté the vegetables for 5 minutes until tender. Remove the pan from the heat. Add the broccoli, oregano, salt, black pepper, Tabasco, and parsley and stir to combine. Beat the egg whites until they form stiff peaks, then fold them gently into the broccoli mixture just until blended. Transfer the batter to the 9" × 13" pan, and gently smooth the top. Mix together the Asiago and bread crumbs and sprinkle the mixture over the frittata. Sprinkle the top with paprika and bake for 30 minutes. Let the frittata cool a bit and cut it into 36 portions.

May be served warm or at room temperature.

Nutritional Analysis

Per Serving

Calories (kcal)	49.0	Cholesterol (mg)	4.0
Total Fat (g)	1.7	Dietary Fiber (g)	1.8
Saturated Fat (g)	0.9	% Calories from Fat	18.6
Monounsaturated Fat (g)	0.1	Vitamin C (mg)	24.0
Polyunsaturated Fat (g)	0.1	Vitamin A (i.u.)	1,130.0

Bruschetta Provençale

This dish is an Italian classic with a French accent and takes minutes to prepare.
It is also wonderful when used as a pasta sauce for 12 ounces
of pasta (makes 4 to 6 servings).

Makes 12 servings

1 28-ounce can plum tomatoes, drained

½ cup chopped fresh basil

1½ teaspoons chopped anchovy fillets (2)

4 kalamata olives, pitted

1 tablespoon capers, drained

3 cloves garlic, minced

1 teaspoon dried oregano

2 tablespoons olive oil

¼ teaspoon salt

¼ teaspoon pepper

1 12-ounce baguette, cut in 36 slices

Coarsely chop the tomatoes and drain them again. Combine the tomatoes with the remaining ingredients, except the bread. Let the mixture set for at least 1 hour to allow the flavors to develop.

Preheat the oven to 350°F.

Toast the bread slices in the oven for 10 minutes. Serve the bruschetta over the toast.

Nutritional Analysis

Per Serving

Calories (kcal)	117.2	Cholesterol (mg)	1.0
Total Fat (g)	3.5	Dietary Fiber (g)	1.5
Saturated Fat (g)	0.5	% Calories from Fat	26.7
Monounsaturated Fat (g)	2.2	Vitamin C (mg)	11.0
Polyunsaturated Fat (g)	0.5	Vitamin A (i.u.)	658.0

CHEESE AND CHILI BEAN DIP

This is a hearty yet low-fat version of a favorite dip. Serve it at your Super Bowl party. It's also terrific in a burrito.

Makes 8 servings

1 16-ounce can vegetarian refried beans

4 ounces grated mozzarella cheese, part skim

3 scallions, chopped

⅓ cup canned, diced chilies

1½ teaspoons chili powder

½ teaspoon ground cumin

½ teaspoon fresh lime juice

½ cup nonfat yogurt

Mix all the ingredients except the yogurt, and gently heat the mixture in a saucepan for several minutes, until the cheese is melted and the dip is well blended. Remove the pan from the heat, add the yogurt and stir to combine.

The dip may be served at room temperature, but it is especially good when heated and served warm with Baked Tortilla Chips (see Index) or raw vegetables.

Nutritional Analysis

Per Serving

Calories (kcal)	101.8	Cholesterol (mg)	8.0
Total Fat (g)	3.1	Dietary Fiber (g)	3.3
Saturated Fat (g)	1.6	% Calories from Fat	27.3
Monounsaturated Fat (g)	0.7	Vitamin C (mg)	13.0
Polyunsaturated Fat (g)	0.1	Vitamin A (i.u.)	318.0

CRAB CROSTINI

This appetizer is as elegant as it is simple, yet easy enough to make as "everyday" sandwiches. (Canned crab can be used, but skip the salt in the recipe.)

Makes 8 servings

8 ounces crab meat, broken up with a fork

⅓ cup chopped scallion

1 tablespoon mayonnaise

1 tablespoon low-fat (1%) buttermilk

2 tablespoons chopped fresh parsley

2 tablespoons chopped fresh chives

1 tablespoon fresh lime juice

1 tablespoon fresh lemon juice

2 teaspoons Dijon mustard

3 tablespoons grated Asiago cheese

¼ teaspoon salt

¼ teaspoon white pepper

1 8-ounce baguette, cut in 32 slices

Preheat the broiler. Line a baking sheet with foil.

Combine all the ingredients except the baguette, and mix well. Spread the mixture on the baguette slices and place them in a single layer on the baking sheet. Broil the crostini for 4 to 5 minutes, about 4 inches from the heat source, until they're golden brown.

Nutritional Analysis

Per Serving

Calories (kcal)	139.5	Cholesterol (mg)	28.0
Total Fat (g)	4.3	Dietary Fiber (g)	1.0
Saturated Fat (g)	1.4	% Calories from Fat	27.8
Monounsaturated Fat (g)	0.8	Vitamin C (mg)	6.0
Polyunsaturated Fat (g)	1.0	Vitamin A (i.u.)	154.0

CROSTINI OF PORCINI MUSHROOMS WITH MADEIRA

Try this sauce on a baked potato in place of butter or sour cream.

Makes 6 servings

1 4-ounce baguette, cut in 18 slices

2 ounces dried porcini mushrooms

1½ cups hot water

1½ tablespoons butter

¼ cup minced shallot

¼ cup Madeira

¼ cup low-sodium chicken broth

½ teaspoon salt

⅛ teaspoon pepper

⅛ teaspoon sugar

½ cup finely chopped fresh parsley

Preheat the oven to 350°F.

Toast the baguette slices in the oven on a baking sheet for 10 minutes, or until they're crisp.

Soak the mushrooms in the hot water for 30 minutes. Drain the mushrooms through a coffee filter or cheesecloth, reserving 1 cup of the liquid. Squeeze the mushrooms dry, blot them with paper towels, and chop them.

Melt the butter in a medium-size saucepan and sauté the shallot for 5 minutes over medium-low heat. Add the mushrooms, reduce the heat to low, and cook the mixture for 5 minutes. Add the Madeira, broth, mushroom liquid, salt, pepper, and sugar and stir to combine. Bring the mixture to a boil, then reduce the heat and simmer the contents for 12 minutes, or until almost all of the liquid evaporates but the mushrooms are still moist. Remove the pan from the heat and stir in the parsley.

Serve the sauce hot, surrounded by toasted baguette slices.

Nutritional Analysis

Per Serving

Calories (kcal)	122.4	Cholesterol (mg)	8.0
Total Fat (g)	3.6	Dietary Fiber (g)	1.8
Saturated Fat (g)	1.9	% Calories from Fat	26.8
Monounsaturated Fat (g)	1.1	Vitamin C (mg)	8.0
Polyunsaturated Fat (g)	0.3	Vitamin A (i.u.)	866.0

Hot Refried Beans with Cream Cheese

These beans are low in fat and high in fiber.

Makes 8 servings

4 corn tortillas

Salt

1 16-ounce can vegetarian refried beans

¼ cup plus 2 tablespoons light cream cheese

2 cloves garlic, minced

¼ cup chopped yellow onion

1 teaspoon ground cumin

2 tablespoons finely chopped fresh cilantro, plus additional chopped cilantro for garnish

Baked Tortilla Chips

Preheat the oven to 350°F. Coat a baking sheet with cooking spray.

Cut the tortillas into eight triangles each and place them in a single layer on the baking sheet. Spray the chips lightly with cooking spray, then sprinkle them lightly with salt. Bake the chips for 10 minutes.

Hot Bean Dip

Combine the beans, the 2 tablespoons cream cheese, the garlic, onion, cumin, and the 2 tablespoons cilantro. Place the mixture in a nonstick pan and cook for 10 minutes over medium-high heat, stirring several times to incorporate the crusty bottom into the rest of the beans.

Transfer the hot bean dip to a small serving plate with sides. Place dollops of the remaining ¼ cup cream cheese on top of the dip, sprinkle it with the remaining cilantro, and serve the hot dip with the tortilla chips.

Nutritional Analysis

Per Serving

Calories (kcal)	105.8	Cholesterol (mg)	6.0
Total Fat (g)	2.7	Dietary Fiber (g)	3.8
Saturated Fat (g)	1.2	% Calories from Fat	23.4
Monounsaturated Fat (g)	0.6	Vitamin C (mg)	3.0
Polyunsaturated Fat (g)	0.2	Vitamin A (i.u.)	114.0

Hummus

This is a classic Middle Eastern food with half the usual amount of oil.
Try it as a dip for raw vegetables. Hummus is also a great sandwich filling
with slices of cucumber, tomato, and red onion.

Makes 12 servings

½ cup sesame seeds

2 tablespoons olive oil

6 cloves garlic, minced

2 15-ounce cans garbanzo
  beans, drained

¾ cup fresh lemon juice

1 teaspoon salt

¼ teaspoon white pepper

2 tablespoons water

20 ounces pita bread (12 slices)

Toast the sesame seeds in a frying pan over medium-low heat for about 3 minutes, shaking the pan often to prevent burning, until the seeds crackle and turn a light golden brown. Let the seeds cool, then place them in a food processor with the olive oil and grind the mixture to a paste. Add the remaining ingredients except the bread, and process the mixture until it's smooth.

Serve the hummus as a dip with the pita bread.

Nutritional Analysis

Per Serving

Calories (kcal)	237.6	Cholesterol (mg)	0.0
Total Fat (g)	6.2	Dietary Fiber (g)	2.6
Saturated Fat (g)	0.9	% Calories from Fat	23.3
Monounsaturated Fat (g)	3.0	Vitamin C (mg)	9.0
Polyunsaturated Fat (g)	1.9	Vitamin A (i.u.)	14.0

LEMON AND CHIVE DIP

This versatile dip may also be enjoyed on baked potatoes, vegetables, seafood, or salad. It can be a low-fat substitute for sour cream or mayonnaise.

Makes 8 servings

1 cup low-fat (1%) cottage cheese

½ cup nonfat yogurt

½ cup part-skim ricotta cheese

¼ cup finely chopped fresh chives

¼ cup finely chopped fresh parsley

2 tablespoons fresh lemon juice

1½ teaspoons lemon zest

1 teaspoon salt

½ teaspoon white pepper

1 teaspoon water

Combine all the ingredients with a wire whisk. Use the mixture as a dip with raw vegetables.

Nutritional Analysis

Per Serving

Calories (kcal)	52.1	Cholesterol (mg)	6.0
Total Fat (g)	1.6	Dietary Fiber (g)	0.2
Saturated Fat (g)	1.0	% Calories from Fat	27.0
Monounsaturated Fat (g)	0.5	Vitamin C (mg)	6.0
Polyunsaturated Fat (g)	0.0	Vitamin A (i.u.)	241.0

Lox and Melon with Chives

Simplicity is the key with this recipe, which illustrates how a few top-quality ingredients can be all that are needed for an excellent dish. A pepper grinder at the table is a nice touch here.

Makes 4 servings

1 pound honeydew melon, peeled and sliced

4 ounces thinly sliced lox

3 tablespoons chopped fresh chives

Freshly ground black pepper

8 lemon slices

Divide the melon among four plates. Top each with a slice of lox. Sprinkle with chives. Season to taste with pepper. Place two lemon slices on each plate and serve.

Nutritional Analysis

Per Serving

Calories (kcal)	62.7	Cholesterol (mg)	7.0
Total Fat (g)	1.4	Dietary Fiber (g)	0.9
Saturated Fat (g)	0.3	% Calories from Fat	16.3
Monounsaturated Fat (g)	0.6	Vitamin C (mg)	42.0
Polyunsaturated Fat (g)	0.3	Vitamin A (i.u.)	160.0

MUSHROOM PÂTÉ

Try this as a sandwich spread, instead of mayonnaise. Or serve the pâté with grilled vegetables—delicious, much more interesting than mayonnaise and a small fraction of the fat!

Makes 10 servings

2 teaspoons olive oil

2 tablespoons finely chopped shallot

2 cloves garlic, minced

1 pound mushrooms, wiped clean and chopped

1 tablespoon balsamic vinegar

2 tablespoons sour cream

2 tablespoons chopped fresh parsley

½ teaspoon salt

¼ teaspoon pepper

30 slices of melba toast

Heat 1 teaspoon of the oil in a large frying pan and sauté the shallot and garlic over medium-low heat for 5 minutes (don't allow them to brown). Add the remaining teaspoon of oil, and raise the heat to medium. Add the mushrooms and vinegar and cook the mixture for 10 minutes, stirring often. (The mushrooms will release moisture. After 10 minutes, the liquid should be evaporated.)

Place the mixture in a food processor and puree until smooth. Let it cool a bit, then add the sour cream, parsley, salt, and pepper, and blend to combine.

Serve the pâté at room temperature with the melba toast.

Nutritional Analysis

Per Serving

Calories (kcal)	83.1	Cholesterol (mg)	1.0
Total Fat (g)	2.1	Dietary Fiber (g)	0.9
Saturated Fat (g)	0.6	% Calories from Fat	22.5
Monounsaturated Fat (g)	0.7	Vitamin C (mg)	3.0
Polyunsaturated Fat (g)	0.3	Vitamin A (i.u.)	282.0

Red Salsa

This salsa can also serve as a salad dressing or as a sauce for chicken, fish, or vegetables. It is a low-fat way to get an abundance of flavor.

Makes 8 servings (2 cups)

1 28-ounce can chopped tomatoes, drained

¼ cup finely chopped scallion

2 tablespoons chopped fresh cilantro

2 tablespoons canned, diced green chilies

1 clove garlic, minced

¼ teaspoon salt

⅛ teaspoon pepper

⅛ teaspoon sugar

1 tablespoon red wine vinegar

Combine all the ingredients. Serve the salsa with Baked Tortilla Chips (See Index.).

Nutritional Analysis

Per Serving

Calories (kcal)	22.6	Cholesterol (mg)	0.0
Total Fat (g)	0.3	Dietary Fiber (g)	1.1
Saturated Fat (g)	0.0	% Calories from Fat	8.7
Monounsaturated Fat (g)	0.0	Vitamin C (mg)	19.0
Polyunsaturated Fat (g)	0.1	Vitamin A (i.u.)	631.0

SALMON MOUSSE WITH BAGUETTES

This dish makes a beautiful presentation yet is low in fat.

Makes 12 servings

1 envelope unflavored gelatin

½ cup boiling water

3 ounces light cream cheese, cut in several pieces

¼ cup part-skim ricotta cheese

1½ tablespoons fresh lemon juice

1 7½-ounce can salmon, drained

⅓ cup chopped fresh chives

¼ teaspoon white pepper

⅓ cup finely chopped bell pepper

10 stuffed green olives, chopped

Paprika

½ cup chopped fresh parsley

12 ounces cherry tomatoes

1 12-ounce baguette, sliced

Coat a 3-cup mold or bowl with cooking spray.

Dissolve the gelatin in the boiling water. Place the gelatin mixture in a food processor with the cream cheese and mix until smooth. Add the ricotta, lemon juice, salmon, chives, white pepper, bell pepper, and olives. Mix until very smooth. Transfer the mixture to the mold. Refrigerate the mousse for several hours, or until it's set.

Unmold the chilled mousse onto a serving plate, sprinkle paprika over the top, garnish the dish with the parsley and tomatoes, and serve with the baguette slices.

Nutritional Analysis

Per Serving

Calories (kcal)	205.9	Cholesterol (mg)	19.0
Total Fat (g)	5.4	Dietary Fiber (g)	2.1
Saturated Fat (g)	2.0	% Calories from Fat	23.6
Monounsaturated Fat (g)	2.0	Vitamin C (mg)	21.0
Polyunsaturated fat (g)	0.9	Vitamin A (i.u.)	578.0

Shrimp Dumplings
with Sun-Dried Tomato Aioli

*These dumplings are simple to prepare. They may be made ahead
and baked just before serving.*

Makes 12 servings

12 ounces cooked shrimp

½ cup finely chopped yellow
onion

4 cloves garlic, minced

2½ teaspoons fresh lemon juice

1½ teaspoons low-sodium soy
sauce

1½ teaspoons cornstarch

¼ teaspoon plus ⅛ teaspoon
white pepper

1 egg white, lightly beaten

12 ounces wonton wrappers
(approximately 56)

2 quarts low-sodium chicken
broth

1½ tablespoons sun-dried
tomatoes (not oil-packed)

1 6-ounce potato, peeled and
cooked

½ cup low-fat (1%) milk

2 tablespoons mayonnaise

1½ tablespoons chopped fresh
basil

¼ teaspoon sugar

¼ teaspoon salt

Shrimp Dumplings

Make the filling by mixing the shrimp, onion, one-half of the garlic, 1½ teaspoons of the lemon juice, the soy sauce, cornstarch, and the ¼ teaspoon
white pepper in a food processor until the mixture is smooth. Add the egg
white and process until well combined.

Place 1 teaspoon of the filling in the center of each wonton wrapper. Moisten
the edges with water, then fold the wonton into a triangle, pressing the edges
together and pressing out the air. Moisten the three points, then fold them
together into a square shape.

Preheat the oven to 400°F. In a medium-size saucepan bring the broth to a
boil over medium heat, then add a few of the dumplings. When the broth
returns to a boil, lower the heat to a simmer and cook for about 2 minutes, or
until the dumplings float to the top. Lift the dumplings out with a slotted
spoon and gently drain them. Repeat until all of the dumplings are cooked.

Place the drained dumplings in a single layer on a baking sheet. Coat both sides of the dumplings lightly with cooking spray. Bake for 3 minutes; turn the dumplings over and bake them for 3 minutes longer.

Serve with Aioli Sauce.

Aioli Sauce

Soak the sun-dried tomatoes in hot water for 15 minutes. Drain the tomatoes, pat them dry, and mince them. Lightly mash the potato with a fork, then mix in the milk until the potato is fluffy. Combine the tomatoes and potato-milk mixture with the remaining garlic, 1 teaspoon lemon juice, ⅛ teaspoon white pepper, the mayonnaise, basil, sugar, and salt.

Nutritional Analysis

Per Serving

Calories (kcal)	177.8	Cholesterol (mg)	59.0
Total Fat (g)	4.5	Dietary Fiber (g)	0.6
Saturated Fat (g)	0.5	% Calories from Fat	19.7
Monounsaturated Fat (g)	0.7	Vitamin C (mg)	7.0
Polyunsaturated Fat (g)	1.3	Vitamin A (i.u.)	105.0

Spinach Dip

This appetizer is a low-fat version of a party favorite.

Makes 8 servings

1 20-ounce package chopped
    frozen spinach, defrosted and
    squeezed dry*

2½ tablespoons mayonnaise

½ cup low-fat (1%) buttermilk

½ teaspoon salt

½ teaspoon pepper

⅓ cup chopped scallion

2 cloves garlic, minced

1 8-ounce baguette, sliced

12 ounces baby carrots

Using a fork, mix the spinach with the mayonnaise until the ingredients are combined and the mixture is fluffy (not compact). Add the buttermilk, salt, pepper, scallion, and garlic and mix until well blended.

Serve the dip with the baguette slices and raw carrots.

---

*The liquid may be saved for soup.

Nutritional Analysis

Per Serving

Calories (kcal)	150.3	Cholesterol (mg)	2.0
Total Fat (g)	5.1	Dietary Fiber (g)	4.1
Saturated Fat (g)	0.8	% Calories from Fat	29.0
Monounsaturated Fat (g)	1.4	Vitamin C (mg)	23.0
Polyunsaturated Fat (g)	2.2	Vitamin A (i.u.)	6,365.0

Sun-Dried Tomato Spread Provençale

Serve this spread with whole-grain crackers for extra "bite."

Makes 12 servings

1 cup (3 ounces) sun-dried tomatoes (not oil-packed)

1½ cups boiling water

2 cloves garlic, minced

¼ cup chopped fresh basil

1 tablespoon capers, drained

6 pitted kalamata olives

1 teaspoon Worcestershire sauce

¼ teaspoon salt

¼ teaspoon pepper

Soak the sun-dried tomatoes in the boiling water for 20 minutes, or until they're soft. Drain the tomatoes, reserving the liquid, and place them in a food processor with the remaining seven ingredients. Blend the mixture well, gradually adding 2 tablespoons of the reserved soaking liquid to make a smooth spread (use more or less, as necessary).

Serve the spread at room temperature on bread or crackers.

Nutritional Analysis

Per Serving

Calories (kcal)	16.1	Cholesterol (mg)	0.0
Total Fat (g)	0.4	Dietary Fiber (g)	0.6
Saturated Fat (g)	0.0	% Calories from Fat	18.4
Monounsaturated Fat (g)	0.2	Vitamin C (mg)	3.0
Polyunsaturated Fat (g)	0.1	Vitamin A (i.u.)	171.0

Tofu-Miso Dip with Lime and Ginger

Use low-fat tofu with approximately 2 grams of fat per 3-ounce serving.

Makes 4 servings

4 ounces low-fat tofu

1 tablespoon vegetable broth
(or chicken broth)

2 tablespoons white miso

1 tablespoon low-sodium
soy sauce

1 teaspoon minced ginger

1 teaspoon fresh lime juice

¼ teaspoon lime zest

1 clove garlic, minced

⅛ teaspoon sugar

Combine all the ingredients in a food processor and process the mixture until it's smooth. Serve it as a dip with raw vegetables, as a sauce for seafood or chicken, or as a dressing for salad or vegetables.

Nutritional Analysis

Per Serving

Calories (kcal)	34.2	Cholesterol (mg)	0.0
Total Fat (g)	1.2	Dietary Fiber (g)	0.7
Saturated Fat (g)	0.2	% Calories from Fat	29.1
Monounsaturated Fat (g)	0.3	Vitamin C (mg)	1.0
Polyunsaturated Fat (g)	0.6	Vitamin A (i.u.)	85.0

Warm Vegetable Caviar

Serve this zesty eggplant appetizer with baguette slices or raw vegetables for dipping. It may be served warm or chilled—and makes a wonderful picnic item. Leftovers freeze well.

Makes 12 servings

¼ cup low-sodium chicken broth

2 cups finely chopped celery

¾ cup finely chopped yellow onion

2 tablespoons olive oil

2 pounds eggplant, peeled and chopped

⅓ cup red wine vinegar

1 tablespoon cider vinegar

1 tablespoon sugar

2 28-ounce cans chopped tomatoes, drained

2 tablespoons tomato paste

6 black kalamata olives, pitted and chopped

1 tablespoon chopped capers, drained

2 chopped anchovy fillets, patted dry

½ teaspoon pepper

1 8-ounce baguette, sliced

Heat the broth in a large frying pan. Add the celery and onion and sauté the vegetables over medium heat for 15 minutes, stirring occasionally. Remove the vegetables from the pan and set them aside. Add the olive oil to the pan, then add the eggplant and sauté the eggplant over medium heat for 5 minutes, stirring often. Return the onion and celery to the pan along with the remaining ingredients, except the baguette. Simmer the contents, uncovered, for 45 minutes, stirring occasionally. Allow the mixture to cool a bit, then chop it in a food processor to medium consistency (don't puree). The caviar may be reheated gently if desired.

While the caviar is cooking, preheat the oven to 350°F and toast the baguette slices for 5 minutes. Serve the toasted baguette slices with the warm caviar.

Nutritional Analysis

Per Serving

Calories (kcal)	113.0	Cholesterol (mg)	1.0
Total Fat (g)	3.4	Dietary Fiber (g)	3.1
Saturated Fat (g)	0.5	% Calories from Fat	25.6
Monounsaturated Fat (g)	2.1	Vitamin C (mg)	9.0
Polyunsaturated Fat (g)	0.5	Vitamin A (i.u.)	360.0

WHOLE BLACK BEAN DIP WITH SALSA

This bean dip has a robust texture and zesty flavor. It is low in fat and calories.

Makes 6 servings

2 teaspoons canola oil	½ cup salsa
½ cup chopped yellow onion	½ teaspoon ground cumin
2 cloves garlic, minced	½ cup (2 ounces) grated
1 15-ounce can black beans, drained	mozzarella cheese, part skim
	¼ cup chopped fresh cilantro
1 cup chopped tomato	1 teaspoon fresh lime juice

Heat the oil in a medium-size skillet, add the onion and garlic, and sauté the vegetables over medium-low heat for 5 minutes, or until they're softened (don't allow them to brown). Add the beans, tomato, salsa, and cumin, raise the heat to medium-high, and cook, stirring often, for 8 minutes, or until most of the liquid has evaporated. Remove the pan from the heat and add the remaining ingredients, stirring to combine.

Serve the dip warm or at room temperature with Baked Tortilla Chips (See Index.).

Nutritional Analysis

Per Serving

Calories (kcal)	85.2	Cholesterol (mg)	3.0
Total Fat (g)	2.0	Dietary Fiber (g)	2.9
Saturated Fat (g)	0.7	% Calories from Fat	20.6
Monounsaturated Fat (g)	0.4	Vitamin C (mg)	7.0
Polyunsaturated Fat (g)	0.6	Vitamin A (i.u.)	256.0

Soups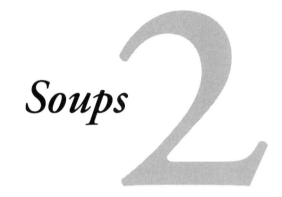

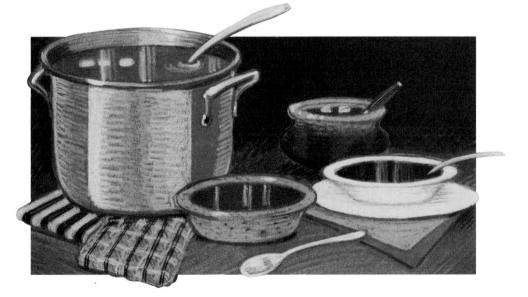

Clear, creamy, or crunchy; sweet or spicy; hot or cold—soup can be fashioned to please every appetite. This wonderful food has been praised for its soothing effects, both the physical and psychological: chicken soup for the sniffles, tomato soup for the blues. The word "soup" itself conjures up images of steamy nourishment, good sustenance, and pleasant dining. Every nationality boasts its favorites, from miso, minestrone, and gazpacho to bouillabaisse, Scotch broth, and borscht.

Soup can be the perfect food on a cancer risk-reduction eating plan. Many varieties of soup in this chapter are low in fat and feature vegetables rich in beta-carotene and vitamin C; cruciferous vegetables; lean meats; poultry and fish; fibrous whole grains; pastas and potatoes; and chemical-free broths and stocks.

If you are a cook with little or no soup-making experience, you will discover that most soups are very simple to prepare. They can be made ahead of time in large quantities and frozen in small containers for quick suppers or hot lunches. There is nothing like homemade soup—and once you begin to make your own, you will never be able to go back to the packaged or canned variety. The clarity of taste and texture in homemade soup is incomparable.

Beginning with the basics, the foundation of any good soup is the broth, which is also called stock, consommé, or bouillon. In this chapter we have included recipes for easy beef, chicken, fish, and vegetable broths.

The success of a good broth depends on the quality and freshness of the ingredients: fresh chicken, meat, and fish; fine herbs such as parsley, thyme, sage, and bay leaf. To ensure the quality of broth, it is vital to adhere to proper cooking temperatures and time (see "Cooking Methods" at the end of this chapter introduction).

All of the broths in this chapter can be served as soups in their original form. Or you can incorporate your own touches—such as chopped scallion, lemon zest, shredded ginger, slivers of lean meat or poultry, fresh parsley, or a sprinkling of grated cheese—for some interesting variations. Add some cooked rice or pasta to the broth with a bit of Parmesan cheese before serving.

Make batches of the assorted broths, and freeze them in small containers for future use. Throughout this book various recipes call for small amounts of broth to moisten a particular dish. A simple way to have a small amount available is to pour homemade broth into ice cube trays; simply defrost single cubes as needed.

We have also included canned commercial broth in some recipes because it is impractical for many cooks to take the time to make homemade broths. If you use canned or commercial broth, select the low-fat, low-sodium variety.

We have tried to include a selection of soups that would satisfy every palate. You'll find our version of some classics such as Gazpacho with Lime Cream, Lentil Soup, and Minestrone with Sweet Potatoes. Soups boasting a wealth of vitamin-rich vegetables include Cream of Broccoli, Roasted Sweet Potato and Onion, and Spinach Soup.

Many soups are hearty and filling meals in themselves. Entree soups include Black Bean Soup with Tomatillos, Chili-Cheese Potato Soup, and Chicken Gumbo. Serve these with a salad and fresh hot bread.

Bread and soup are a natural combination. The word *soup* is actually derived from the Germanic word *sop*—the bread over which the watery soup was poured. In some parts of France, *le soupe* still refers to the piece of bread that accompanies the broth or soup. Bread and soup from the earliest times have always been inseparable. In Chapter 9, "Sweet and Savory Bakery," you will find many varieties of delicious breads that need little or no butter or margarine to taste great. Try Corn Bread or Fresh Herb Muffins with some of these hearty soups.

For the creative cook with limited time, there is no end to the kinds of soups you can make simply by searching the refrigerator for leftover vegetables such as cauliflower, broccoli, or spinach. Heat the vegetable over a low flame; add cooked potato for thickening. When the mixture is heated through (about 5 minutes), whirl it through a blender or food processor. Return it to the pot and heat it a few more minutes. Garnish the dish with a sprinkling of Parmesan cheese and cracked fresh pepper. This is "instant" homemade soup, delicious for a chilly evening's meal or a quick and satisfying lunch. Serve your creation with Mini Scallion-Cheese Scones or Irish Soda Bread.

The soups in this chapter abound with a wealth of healthful vegetables— cabbage, broccoli, spinach, green peppers, sweet potatoes, winter squash—and provide an excellent source of vitamins. Since the vegetables are cooked and served in the same liquid, no vitamins are drained off.

All of our soups are lower in fat than the standard varieties, so you can have a second cup without feeling guilty. "Soup's on!" won't mean "pounds on" for you with these recipes.

Cooking Methods

The success of good soup depends on the quality of the broth. When you're making stock or broth, the ingredients should be simmered. Vegetables begin to disintegrate when cooked on high heat, and this will make the liquid murky. During the first half hour of cooking, check vegetable broth at frequent intervals to make sure the liquid is not boiling. Beef, chicken, and fish broths, however, need to be boiled in order to seal the flavors. After the broth is cooked through for flavor, strain the liquid through a mesh strainer or two layers of cheesecloth. This will yield a delicate tasting and clear stock. Then, if you want a stronger taste, boil the stock down to concentrate the liquid.

To shorten cooking time, chop meats and vegetables into small pieces; they will yield flavor faster (see Easy Beef Broth). This fast broth will have a lighter flavor because you don't use the bones and trimmings (which make a stronger-tasting stock because of the longer cooking time needed to release their gelatin).

If any fat remains in the broth after straining, chill the liquid, then skim the hardened fat from the top. If you are in a hurry, gently skim the top of the broth with a paper towel. If you use packaged or regular canned broth, do not add any salt to the recipe and remember to chill the can first so that you can easily skim the fat.

Creamed soups, by definition, are a puree of ingredients to which heavy cream—or sometimes a roux of butter and flour—has been added to thicken the dish. Obviously there is no place for heavy cream on a cancer risk-reduction eating plan. But you don't need that kind of cream to get the desired taste and consistency that creamed soups boast. Just try our Cream of Broccoli Soup, Creamy Sweet Potato Soup, or Apple-Squash Soup with Chive Sour Cream.

You can also use potato as a base for any creamy vegetable soup. Both pureed potato and boiled potato work very well as soup thickeners.

A last word on cooking soup: never overboil—the ingredients will turn to mush. You want vegetables to be soft but not overcooked. The harder or denser the consistency of the vegetable (carrots, turnips, etc.), the longer they will take to cook. If hard vegetables are mixed with soft vegetables such as peas or leafy vegetables such as spinach, the dense vegetables should be put into the pot first. Then the others should be added just a few minutes before the soup is done.

And remember—when you're reheating soup, it should be simmered!

APPLE-SQUASH SOUP
WITH CHIVE SOUR CREAM

The inherent sweetness of the apple and squash in this recipe is balanced by the garlic, lemon juice, and spices. The squash is rich in beta-carotene.

Makes 8 servings

2 tablespoons olive oil

1 cup chopped yellow onion

1 clove garlic, minced

2 10-ounce packages frozen butternut squash, defrosted

1 quart low-fat chicken broth

2 cups peeled, chopped apple

2 teaspoons fresh lemon juice

1 teaspoon dried thyme

½ teaspoon salt

¾ teaspoon white pepper

1 cup low-fat (1%) milk

½ cup light sour cream

2 tablespoons chopped fresh chives

Heat the oil in a large saucepan over medium-low heat. Add the onion and garlic and sauté the vegetables for 10 minutes. Add the squash, broth, apple, lemon juice, thyme, salt, and ½ teaspoon of the pepper and bring to a boil. Reduce the heat and simmer the contents for 20 minutes.

Puree the soup in a blender or food processor, then return it to the pan. Stir in the milk and heat the soup for 10 more minutes.

Top each serving with a tablespoon of the sour cream mixed with the chives and remaining ¼ teaspoon pepper.

Nutritional Analysis

Per Serving

Calories (kcal)	135.2	Cholesterol (mg)	2.0
Total Fat (g)	4.2	Dietary Fiber (g)	2.2
Saturated Fat (g)	0.7	% Calories from Fat	23.3
Monounsaturated Fat (g)	2.6	Vitamin C (mg)	9.0
Polyunsaturated Fat (g)	0.4	Vitamin A (i.u.)	4,189.0

Black Bean Soup with Tomatillos

This hot, colorful soup is wonderfully festive with a cool, white sour cream mixture in the center of each bowl, dotted with cilantro as a garnish. It has only 12.3 percent calories from fat and provides 20.1 grams of fiber per serving.

Makes 8 servings

2 tablespoons canola oil

2 cups chopped yellow onion

3 cloves garlic, minced

2 teaspoons chili powder

½ teaspoon red pepper flakes

½ teaspoon salt

1 pound new potatoes, unpeeled and chopped

3 carrots, unpeeled and chopped

1 30-ounce can black beans, drained

1 24-ounce can tomatillos, drained

5 cups low-sodium chicken broth

1½ teaspoons fresh lemon juice

1½ teaspoons fresh lime juice

4 tablespoons sour cream

4 tablespoons nonfat yogurt

4 tablespoons chopped fresh cilantro

Heat the oil in a large pot over medium-low heat. Add the onion, garlic, chili powder, red pepper flakes, and salt and cook the mixture for 10 minutes. Add the potato, carrot, beans, tomatillos, and broth and bring the contents to a boil. Reduce the heat, partially cover the pot, and simmer the soup until the vegetables are tender, about 45 minutes. Add the lemon and lime juices.

Combine the sour cream and yogurt and place a dollop in the center of each serving of hot soup. Sprinkle the cilantro on top.

Nutritional Analysis

Per Serving

Calories (kcal)	513.3	Cholesterol (mg)	3.0
Total Fat (g)	7.6	Dietary Fiber (g)	20.1
Saturated Fat (g)	1.8	% Calories from Fat	12.3
Monounsaturated Fat (g)	1.4	Vitamin C (mg)	25.0
Polyunsaturated Fat (g)	2.8	Vitamin A (i.u.)	7,163.0

CHICKEN GUMBO

Low in fat, yet hearty and filling, this soup is a meal in itself.

Makes 8 servings (4 as an entree)

1 pound boned and skinned chicken breast halves, cut in bite-size pieces

3 cups water

2 cups low-sodium chicken broth

2 cloves garlic, minced

½ teaspoon red pepper flakes

1 cup chopped yellow onion

1 bay leaf

½ teaspoon dried sage

1 teaspoon dried thyme

2 cups sliced okra, fresh or frozen

2 cups chopped tomato

2 cups corn, fresh or frozen

1 teaspoon salt

½ teaspoon pepper

2 cups brown rice

2 tablespoons butter

2 tablespoons flour

Rinse the chicken and place it in a large pot. Cover the chicken with the water and 1 cup of the broth and bring the liquid to a boil. Skim off the foam with a slotted spoon, then add the garlic, red pepper flakes, onion, bay leaf, sage, and thyme. Cover the pot and let the soup simmer for 20 minutes. Add the okra, tomatoes, and corn. Cover the pot and continue simmering for 20 minutes. Add the salt and pepper.

While the soup is simmering, cook the rice according to the package directions (takes about 40 minutes).

Melt the butter in a small pan, add the flour, and stir over medium heat until the roux is dark golden brown and bubbly. Add the remaining cup of chicken broth and bring the liquid to a boil. Reduce the heat and whisk the contents until smooth. Add this mixture to the soup pot and stir to combine.

Serve the gumbo in large soup bowls with a scoop of the rice.

Nutritional Analysis

Per Serving

Calories (kcal)	336.4	Cholesterol (mg)	41.0
Total Fat (g)	5.6	Dietary Fiber (g)	3.7
Saturated Fat (g)	2.3	% Calories from Fat	14.4
Monounsaturated Fat (g)	3.1	Vitamin C (mg)	21.0
Polyunsaturated Fat (g)	1.0	Vitamin A (i.u.)	794.0

CHILI-CHEESE POTATO SOUP

This soup is low in fat and high in beta-carotene.

Makes 12 generous servings

1½ tablespoons olive oil

2 pounds leeks (white part only), chopped

1½ cups chopped yellow onion

4 pounds new potatoes, unpeeled, scrubbed, and chopped

1 pound carrots, unpeeled, scrubbed, and chopped

3 quarts low-sodium chicken broth

½ teaspoon salt

1½ teaspoon ground cumin

½ teaspoon white pepper

1 4-ounce can diced green chilies

4 ounces extra-sharp shredded cheddar cheese

1 cup low-fat (1%) milk

1 teaspoon red pepper flakes (optional)

¼ teaspoon cayenne (optional)

1 cup finely chopped fresh parsley

Heat the oil in a large pot over medium-low heat. Add the leek and onion and sauté for 10 minutes. Add the potato, carrot, broth, salt, cumin, and pepper and bring the mixture to a boil. Stir, reduce the heat, and simmer the contents, partially covered, for 45 minutes.

With a slotted spoon or small strainer, transfer the vegetables to a food processor and puree them (in two or three batches if necessary). Return the pureed vegetables to the pot, and add the chilies, cheese, milk, red pepper flakes, and cayenne and stir the mixture to blend the ingredients. Heat the soup on low until the cheese is melted and the soup is hot.

Sprinkle each serving with the parsley.

Nutritional Analysis

Per Serving

Calories (kcal)	217.0	Cholesterol (mg)	11.0
Total Fat (g)	5.5	Dietary Fiber (g)	4.1
Saturated Fat (g)	2.4	% Calories from Fat	19.1
Monounsaturated Fat (g)	2.2	Vitamin C (mg)	49.0
Polyunsaturated Fat (g)	0.4	Vitamin A (i.u.)	9,977.0

Chilled Cucumber and Dill Soup

*This is a wonderful soup for spring or summer. It's a special addition
to a picnic or brunch and makes a light summer meal
along with whole-grain bread and some fruit for dessert.*

Makes 4 servings (1 quart)

2 pounds cucumbers (about 2
large)

1 scallion, minced

½ cup nonfat yogurt

1½ cups low-fat (1%)
buttermilk

3 tablespoons sour cream

1 clove garlic, minced

1 teaspoon balsamic vinegar

1 teaspoon dried dill

1 teaspoon salt

¼ teaspoon white pepper

⅛ teaspoon sugar

Peel the cucumbers and cut each in half lengthwise. With a small spoon,
scrape the seeds out from the center. Finely chop the cucumber and combine
it with the remaining ingredients. Cover the bowl and let the soup sit for
1 hour to allow the flavor to develop. Refrigerate the soup for 2 hours before
serving.

Nutritional Analysis

Per Serving

Calories (kcal)	118.0	Cholesterol (mg)	9.0
Total Fat (g)	3.5	Dietary Fiber (g)	2.7
Saturated Fat (g)	2.0	% Calories from Fat	25.1
Monounsaturated Fat (g)	0.9	Vitamin C (mg)	20.0
Polyunsaturated Fat (g)	0.3	Vitamin A (i.u.)	700.0

Chilled Fresh Tomato Soup

Easy, quick, low in calories and fat, this soup is perfect for lunch on a hot summer day.

Makes 6 servings

2 pounds tomatoes

2 tablespoons chopped fresh basil

2 tablespoons finely chopped yellow onion

2 cups chicken broth

2 teaspoons sugar

½ teaspoon salt

½ teaspoon white pepper

Dip the tomatoes in boiling water for 30 seconds, then peel and seed them. Immediately place them in a bowl of ice-cold water; when they're cool enough to handle, peel the skin off with a knife (it should slip off easily); cut each tomato in half along its equator and squeeze the seeds out, reserving as much liquid as possible. Cut the cores from the tomatoes, then quarter them and whirl the pieces in a food processor (in batches, if necessary) until they're well pureed.

In a large bowl combine the tomato puree with the remaining ingredients and the reserved juice. Place the bowl in the refrigerator for several hours to allow the flavors to develop.

Serve the soup slightly chilled or at room temperature.

Nutritional Analysis

Per Serving

Calories (kcal)	92.3	Cholesterol (mg)	1.0
Total Fat (g)	1.3	Dietary Fiber (g)	3.1
Saturated Fat (g)	0.3	% Calories from Fat	11.5
Monounsaturated Fat (g)	0.4	Vitamin C (mg)	53.0
Polyunsaturated Fat (g)	0.4	Vitamin A (i.u.)	1,738.0

Chinese Mushroom and Tofu Soup with Greens

This soup makes a terrific beginning to an Asian meal or, with the addition of leftover poultry or meat, a simple but complete meal in itself.

Makes 6 servings

1 ounce dried shiitake mushrooms

1½ quarts chicken broth

⅛ teaspoon pepper

1½ cups chopped watercress

1½ cups chopped Chinese cabbage

2 tablespoons cornstarch

2 tablespoons sherry

1 scallion, sliced

6 ounces tofu, drained

¼ teaspoon salt

Soak the mushrooms in 1 cup of water for 30 minutes, then drain them, reserving the liquid. Discard any tough stems, then slice the mushrooms.

Bring the broth to a boil in a large pot. Add the pepper, watercress, and cabbage. Simmer the mixture for 3 minutes.

Stir the cornstarch and 2 tablespoons of water together. Bring the soup back to a boil and add the cornstarch mixture, stirring constantly until it is incorporated into the soup. Simmer for 1 minute. Stir in the mushrooms, the reserved liquid, and the remaining ingredients. Heat the soup thoroughly, but don't boil it.

Serve hot.

Nutritional Analysis

Per Serving

Calories (kcal)	80.9	Cholesterol (mg)	0.0
Total Fat (g)	1.5	Dietary Fiber (g)	1.9
Saturated Fat (g)	0.2	% Calories from Fat	11.5
Monounsaturated Fat (g)	0.3	Vitamin C (mg)	17.0
Polyunsaturated Fat (g)	0.8	Vitamin A (i.u.)	947.0

CREAM OF BROCCOLI SOUP

This recipe is high in both vitamin C and beta-carotene.

Makes 6 servings

3 cups broccoli florets	3 cups low-fat (1%) milk
2 cups low-fat chicken broth	½ teaspoon salt
1 tablespoon butter	¼ teaspoon white pepper
½ cup chopped yellow onion	¼ teaspoon paprika
1 tablespoon flour	¼ teaspoon celery seed

Finely chop the broccoli florets. Bring the broth to a boil in a medium-size saucepan. Add the broccoli, reduce the heat, and simmer, covered, for 10 minutes. Set the pan aside but do not drain the liquid.

Melt the butter in a large pan over medium heat, add the onion, and sauté until the onion is soft, about 5 minutes. Blend in the flour and cook until thickened. Add the milk, then raise the heat and incorporate the milk into the onion-flour mixture. Add the broccoli and the cooking broth and all the remaining ingredients. Stir to combine and simmer gently over low heat until the soup is hot.

Nutritional Analysis

Per Serving

Calories (kcal)	106.8	Cholesterol (mg)	10.0
Total Fat (g)	3.5	Dietary Fiber (g)	2.6
Saturated Fat (g)	2.0	% Calories from Fat	25.3
Monounsaturated Fat (g)	1.0	Vitamin C (mg)	55.0
Polyunsaturated Fat (g)	0.3	Vitamin A (i.u.)	1,482.0

CREAMY SWEET POTATO SOUP

This brightly colored soup is rich and creamy and takes only minutes to make. The flavor and texture belie the fact that it has only 8.3 percent calories from fat. In addition, it contains 45 percent of the recommended daily allowance of vitamin C and 33.4 percent of the RDA of beta-carotene.

Makes 6 servings

1½ pounds sweet potatoes or yams

1 quart low-sodium chicken broth

1 cup chopped yellow onion

3 cloves garlic, minced

1 teaspoon dried savory

½ teaspoon salt

¼ teaspoon white pepper

1½ cups low-fat (1%) milk

¼ cup chopped fresh parsley

Peel the sweet potatoes and coarsely chop them. In a large pot, combine the potatoes with the remaining ingredients except the milk and parsley. Cover the pot and simmer the mixture over medium-low heat for 20 minutes, or until the potatoes are tender.

With a slotted spoon transfer the vegetables to a food processor and puree them until smooth. Return the pureed vegetables to the pot, add the milk, and gently reheat the soup.

Sprinkle each serving with the parsley.

Nutritional Analysis

Per Serving

Calories (kcal)	145.7	Cholesterol (mg)	2.0
Total Fat (g)	1.6	Dietary Fiber (g)	4.1
Saturated Fat (g)	0.6	% Calories from Fat	8.3
Monounsaturated Fat (g)	0.2	Vitamin C (mg)	27.0
Polyunsaturated Fat (g)	0.1	Vitamin A (i.u.)	16,681.0

CREAMY VEGETABLE SOUP

This soup can be served hot or chilled. Make it more elegant by floating a paper-thin slice of lemon on top, adding a dollop of nonfat yogurt, and sprinkling each serving with fresh chives.

Makes 6 servings

1 tablespoon butter

½ pound broccoli florets, chopped fine

½ pound zucchini, sliced

1½ quarts low-fat chicken broth

½ bunch parsley, chopped

½ bunch watercress, chopped

¼ teaspoon salt

¼ teaspoon white pepper

¾ cup nonfat yogurt

Melt the butter in a large pot, add the broccoli, and sauté the broccoli until it's softened, about 10 minutes. Add the zucchini and cook 5 minutes more. Add the broth, parsley, watercress, salt, and pepper. Simmer the contents for 20 minutes uncovered.

Transfer the mixture to a food processor and puree until smooth. Return the pureed mixture to the pot, add the yogurt, and heat gently, whisking to combine.

The soup may be served hot or chilled.

Nutritional Analysis

Per Serving

Calories (kcal)	80.6	Cholesterol (mg)	6.0
Total Fat (g)	2.3	Dietary Fiber (g)	2.2
Saturated Fat (g)	1.2	% Calories from Fat	17.2
Monounsaturated Fat (g)	0.6	Vitamin C (mg)	37.0
Polyunsaturated Fat (g)	0.1	Vitamin A (i.u.)	2,026.0

Easy Beef Broth

This easily made broth is quick enough for the busiest cook. The meat and vegetables left after straining can be used for vegetable-beef soup. The broth may be stored in the freezer for use when needed.

Makes 1 quart (4 1-cup servings)

1 pound beef bottom round or other lean beef

1½ pounds potatoes, unpeeled and chopped

3 cups chopped celery

3 cups chopped carrot

3 cups chopped leek (white part only)

½ teaspoon salt

1 quart cold water

Remove all visible fat from the beef, then cut the meat into small cubes. Place the beef and all the remaining ingredients in a large pan and bring the liquid to a boil. Partly cover the pan and cook the contents on the lowest heat for 1 hour. Strain the broth through a mesh strainer.

Chill the broth and remove the fat from the top.

Nutritional Analysis

Per Serving

Calories (kcal)	222.0	Cholesterol (mg)	70.0
Total Fat (g)	15.4	Dietary Fiber (g)	7.2
Saturated Fat (g)	5.8	% Calories from Fat	9.6
Monounsaturated Fat (g)	6.6	Vitamin C (mg)	48.0
Polyunsaturated Fat (g)	0.8	Vitamin A (i.u.)	2,083.0

EASY CHICKEN BROTH

This recipe not only gives you homemade broth that is much healthier than the commercial varieties, but it also yields poached chicken breasts to use for sandwiches, salads, or an entree (try them with one of the low-fat sauces or condiments in this book). The broth may be stored in the freezer for use when needed.

Makes 1½ quarts (6 1-cup servings)

3 pounds boned and skinned chicken breast halves

2 bay leaves

1 carrot, unpeeled and chopped coarse

2 cloves garlic, minced

2 celery ribs, chopped coarse

4 parsley sprigs

1 teaspoon salt

¼ teaspoon white pepper

5 cups water

Rinse the chicken breasts and put them in a large pot with all the remaining ingredients. Bring the liquid to a boil, skim off the foam, cover the pot, and simmer the contents until the chicken is tender, about 30 minutes. Remove the chicken and save it for another use.

Simmer the liquid and vegetables for an additional 30 minutes (or longer if a stronger flavor is desired), skimming off any foam. Strain the broth through a mesh strainer.

Chill the broth and remove the fat from the top.

Nutritional Analysis

Per Serving

Calories (kcal)	48.0	Cholesterol (mg)	132.0
Total Fat (g)	2.9	Dietary Fiber (g)	0.7
Saturated Fat (g)	0.8	% Calories from Fat	10.6
Monounsaturated Fat (g)	6.8	Vitamin C (mg)	6.0
Polyunsaturated Fat (g)	0.7	Vitamin A (i.u.)	3,154.0

EASY FISH BROTH

*A good fish broth is difficult to find in the market, but this one is simple to make
and has a delicate seafood flavor rather than a strong salt flavor.*

Makes about 1½ quarts (6 1-cup servings)

2 pounds fish bones and
trimmings

1 cup chopped yellow onion

1 clove garlic, halved

1 carrot, unpeeled and chopped
coarse

2 celery ribs, chopped

1 cup white wine

½ cup parsley sprigs

2 bay leaves

3 whole black peppercorns

¼ teaspoon dried thyme

2 quarts water

Place all the ingredients in a stockpot and bring the liquid to a boil. Skim off
any foam that rises to the top. Partially cover the pot and simmer the contents
for 1½ hours. Strain the broth through a mesh strainer.

Chill the broth and remove the fat from the top.

Nutritional Analysis

Per Serving

Calories (kcal)	56.5	Cholesterol (mg)	0.0
Total Fat (g)	0.3	Dietary Fiber (g)	7.3
Saturated Fat (g)	0.1	% Calories from Fat	7.2
Monounsaturated Fat (g)	0.1	Vitamin C (mg)	14.0
Polyunsaturated Fat (g)	0.1	Vitamin A (i.u.)	3,272.0

EASY VEGETABLE BROTH

This recipe is much lower in sodium than commercial vegetarian broths.
The broth may be stored in the freezer for use when needed.

Makes about 2 quarts (8 1-cup servings)

3 cups chopped carrot

1 bunch parsley, chopped coarse

3 cups chopped celery

4 cloves garlic, chopped coarse

2 yellow onions, chopped
  coarse

3 bay leaves

1 teaspoon dried sage

1 teaspoon dried thyme

1 teaspoon salt

½ teaspoon white pepper

2 quarts cold water

2 tablespoons fresh lemon juice

Place all the ingredients in a large pot and bring the liquid to a boil. Reduce the heat, cover the pot, and simmer the contents for 1 hour. Let the mixture cool a bit, then strain it through a mesh strainer, pressing the juices out of the vegetables. Discard the vegetables.

Use this broth in vegetarian dishes or whenever a light broth is desired.

Nutritional Analysis

Per Serving

Calories (kcal)	64.0	Cholesterol (mg)	0.0
Total Fat (g)	0.6	Dietary Fiber (g)	3.5
Saturated Fat (g)	0.1	% Calories from Fat	7.3
Monounsaturated Fat (g)	0.0	Vitamin C (mg)	21.0
Polyunsaturated Fat (g)	0.1	Vitamin A (i.u.)	12,184.0

GAZPACHO WITH LIME CREAM

This Spanish classic is high in beta-carotene.

Makes 8 servings

1 cup low-fat chicken broth

¼ cup sherry vinegar

2 teaspoons olive oil

2 cups tomato sauce

½ cup fresh orange juice

⅛ teaspoon cayenne

1 teaspoon chopped fresh basil

1 large cucumber

¾ cup chopped yellow onion

1 cup chopped green bell pepper

1 28-ounce can tomatoes, drained

2 cloves garlic, minced

3 tablespoons sour cream

5 tablespoons nonfat yogurt

1½ tablespoons fresh lime juice

¼ teaspoon salt

In a serving bowl, combine the broth, vinegar, oil, tomato sauce, orange juice, cayenne, and basil. In a food processor, combine the cucumber, onion, bell pepper, tomatoes, and garlic and chop, leaving some texture—*don't puree.* Add the vegetables to the serving bowl. Chill for several hours to allow flavors to develop.

Mix the sour cream, yogurt, lime juice, and salt. Top each serving of chilled soup with a generous spoonful of the sour cream mixture.

Nutritional Analysis

Per Serving

Calories (kcal)	85.1	Cholesterol (mg)	3.0
Total Fat (g)	2.7	Dietary Fiber (g)	2.5
Saturated Fat (g)	0.9	% Calories from Fat	24.5
Monounsaturated Fat (g)	1.2	Vitamin C (mg)	34.0
Polyunsaturated Fat (g)	0.3	Vitamin A (i.u.)	1,193.0

HOT-AND-SOUR SOUP

The "hot" comes from the pepper, and "sour" from the vinegar. If you like highly seasoned food, you might want to add more vinegar and pepper. The more you add, the spicier and more piquant the soup will be.

Makes 8 servings

2 ounces dried shiitake mushrooms

½ cup bean threads or cellophane noodles (found in the Asian section of the supermarket)

1½ quarts low-fat chicken broth

4 ounces cooked, shredded chicken breast

½ cup grated carrot

¼ cup sliced scallion

½ cup canned water chestnuts, drained and sliced

1 teaspoon soy sauce

1 teaspoon sugar

3 tablespoons red wine vinegar

½ teaspoon pepper

2 tablespoons cornstarch

1 egg, beaten

1 teaspoon sesame oil

8 ounces tofu

½ cup chopped fresh cilantro

Soak the mushrooms and bean threads, separately, in water to cover for 30 minutes. Drain the mushrooms (discarding tough stems) and bean threads.

In a large pot, bring the broth to a boil and add the mushrooms, bean threads, chicken, carrot, scallion, and water chestnuts and simmer the contents for 10 minutes. Add the soy sauce, sugar, vinegar, and pepper and stir. Mix the cornstarch with 2 tablespoons of water. Heat the soup to boiling and add the cornstarch-water mixture. Reduce the heat a bit and stir until the soup is slightly thickened.

Remove the pot from the heat and stir in the egg (the egg will cook completely). Add the sesame oil and tofu and gently heat the soup through. Taste for flavors, adding more vinegar or pepper as desired.

Serve the soup hot, garnished with the cilantro.

Nutritional Analysis

Per Serving

Calories (kcal)	123.3	Cholesterol (mg)	32.0
Total Fat (g)	3.5	Dietary Fiber (g)	1.6
Saturated Fat (g)	0.7	% Calories from Fat	20.3
Monounsaturated Fat (g)	1.1	Vitamin C (mg)	3.0
Polyunsaturated Fat (g)	1.3	Vitamin A (i.u.)	1,826.0

LENTIL SOUP

This soup boasts wonderful taste and 12.9 grams of fiber.

Makes 10 servings

2 tablespoons olive oil

2 cups lentils

1 cup chopped yellow onion

1 cup chopped carrot

¼ cup chopped fresh parsley

2 cloves garlic, minced

½ teaspoon salt

½ teaspoon pepper

½ teaspoon dried thyme

2 quarts low-fat chicken broth

2 cups chopped tomato

2 tablespoons white wine vinegar

Heat the oil in a large pot over medium heat. Add the lentils, onion, carrot, parsley, garlic, salt, pepper, and thyme and sauté for 15 minutes. Add the broth and tomato to the pot and simmer the contents, covered, for 1½ hours. Add the vinegar and simmer 30 minutes longer.

Serve hot.

Nutritional Analysis

Per Serving

Calories (kcal)	190.3	Cholesterol (mg)	0.0
Total Fat (g)	3.3	Dietary Fiber (g)	12.9
Saturated Fat (g)	0.4	% Calories from Fat	13.1
Monounsaturated Fat (g)	2.1	Vitamin C (mg)	16.0
Polyunsaturated Fat (g)	0.5	Vitamin A (i.u.)	3,147.0

Minestrone with Sweet Potatoes

When you add sweet potatoes to this popular soup, the beta-carotene content is incomparable, truly making it a cancer prevention dish.

Makes 6 servings

2 tablespoons olive oil

1 cup chopped yellow onion

1 cup chopped carrot

1 cup chopped celery

2 cloves garlic, minced

3 cups low-sodium chicken broth

2 cups unpeeled, chopped sweet potato

1 teaspoon chopped fresh basil

½ teaspoon salt

½ teaspoon pepper

1 28-ounce can chopped tomatoes, undrained

1 15-ounce can white beans, drained

½ pound washed and chopped Swiss chard

Heat the oil in a large pot over medium heat. Add the onion, carrot, celery, and garlic and sauté the vegetables for 10 minutes. Add the remaining ingredients, except the Swiss chard, to the pot and bring the contents to a boil. Reduce the heat, partially cover the pot, and simmer for 30 minutes. Stir the Swiss chard into the pot and heat the soup for 5 minutes longer, over low heat.

Serve hot.

Nutritional Analysis

Per Serving

Calories (kcal)	162.9	Cholesterol (mg)	0.0
Total Fat (g)	4.0	Dietary Fiber (g)	5.9
Saturated Fat (g)	0.6	% Calories from Fat	19.8
Monounsaturated Fat (g)	2.5	Vitamin C (mg)	32.0
Polyunsaturated Fat (g)	0.5	Vitamin A (i.u.)	9,633.0

POTATO AND LEEK SOUP
WITH GOLDEN VEGETABLES

*This soup could also be served as vichyssoise by pureeing the mixture
to a fine texture, pressing it through a mesh strainer, and serving it
chilled with a sprinkling of fresh chives.*

Makes 8 servings

1½ tablespoons canola oil

1½ tablespoons butter

2 pounds leeks (white part only), chopped

2 pounds potatoes, peeled and chopped

1 small rutabaga, chopped

½ pound carrots, unpeeled, scrubbed, and chopped

1½ quarts low-fat chicken broth

½ teaspoon salt

¼ teaspoon white pepper

1 cup low-fat (1%) milk

½ cup finely chopped fresh parsley

Heat the oil and butter in a large pot over low heat; add the leeks and sauté for 10 minutes. Add the potato, rutabaga, carrot, broth, salt, and pepper to the pot and simmer the contents, partially covered, for 45 minutes. Transfer the mixture to a food processor and puree slightly, leaving some texture (you may need to do this in two batches). Return the puree to the pot, add the milk, and simmer gently until the soup is thoroughly heated.

Serve the soup hot, garnishing each portion with a sprinkling of the parsley.

Nutritional Analysis

Per Serving

Calories (kcal)	182.9	Cholesterol (mg)	7.0
Total Fat (g)	5.3	Dietary Fiber (g)	3.5
Saturated Fat (g)	1.9	% Calories From Fat	22.4
Monounsaturated Fat (g)	1.3	Vitamin C (mg)	34.0
Polyunsaturated Fat (g)	1.7	Vitamin A (i.u.)	7,575.0

Roasted Sweet Potato and Onion Soup

Sweet potatoes are sold under several different names. For this recipe, look for yams. Roasting brings out the sweetness in both the sweet potato and onion. The yogurt–sour cream topping is a wonderful contrast to the natural sweetness of the roasted vegetables.

Makes 6 servings

¼ cup nonfat yogurt

2 tablespoons light sour cream

2 tablespoons chopped Italian flat-leaf parsley

1 clove garlic, minced

1½ pounds sweet potatoes, peeled and sliced

1 medium yellow onion, sliced

4 cups low-fat (1%) milk

½ teaspoon salt

¼ teaspoon white pepper

Preheat the oven to 400°F. Coat a baking sheet with cooking spray.

Combine the yogurt, sour cream, parsley, and garlic. Set the mixture aside as a garnish for the soup.

Place the sweet potatoes in a single layer on the baking sheet. Separate the onion slices into rings and place them on top of the sweet potato. Roast the vegetables for 20 minutes.

Transfer the vegetables to a food processor and process them until smooth. Pour the processed vegetables into a saucepan and add the milk, salt, and pepper. Whisk the mixture to combine the ingredients.

Heat the soup gently and garnish each serving with a tablespoon of the yogurt–sour cream topping.

Nutritional Analysis

Per Serving

Calories (kcal)	180.2	Cholesterol (mg)	9.0
Total Fat (g)	3.0	Dietary Fiber (g)	2.9
Saturated Fat (g)	1.8	% Calories from Fat	15.0
Monounsaturated Fat (g)	0.8	Vitamin C (mg)	24.0
Polyunsaturated Fat (g)	0.2	Vitamin A (i.u.)	16,832.0

SOUTHWEST CORN BISQUE WITH HERB CREAM

This corn bisque is a good example of an easily prepared soup that involves no sautéing yet is delicious, elegant, contemporary, and low in fat.

Makes 6 servings

3 cloves garlic, minced

3 cups corn, fresh or frozen (don't use canned corn—the taste isn't delicate enough)

4½ cups low-fat chicken broth

¾ cup chopped yellow onion

⅓ cup chopped carrot

⅓ cup chopped celery

1 tablespoon canned, diced green chilies

1½ cups low-fat (1%) milk

3 tablespoons light sour cream

6 tablespoons nonfat yogurt

3 tablespoons finely chopped fresh parsley

1 tablespoon chopped fresh basil

1 tablespoon chopped fresh cilantro

½ teaspoon ground cumin

½ teaspoon salt

In a large pot, combine the garlic, corn, broth, onion, carrot, celery, and chilies. Bring the mixture to a boil, reduce the heat, and simmer the contents for 1 hour. Strain the mixture through a mesh strainer, pressing hard to extract the juices from the vegetables. Discard the vegetables.

Transfer the liquid to a clean pot, add the milk, and simmer the soup for 5 minutes.

Combine the sour cream, yogurt, herbs, and spices. Swirl a spoonful of the sour cream–herb mixture into the center of each serving of soup.

Nutritional Analysis

Per Serving

Calories (kcal)	131.0	Cholesterol (mg)	3.0
Total Fat (g)	1.9	Dietary Fiber (g)	2.8
Saturated Fat (g)	0.6	% Calories from Fat	10.2
Monounsaturated Fat (g)	0.5	Vitamin C (mg)	10.0
Polyunsaturated Fat (g)	0.5	Vitamin A (i.u.)	2,007.0

SPINACH SOUP

*Popeye never tasted soup this good! Just look at
the beta-carotene and vitamin C content.*

Makes 6 servings

2 cups low-fat (1%) milk

5 cups low-fat chicken broth

2 10-ounce packages frozen
chopped spinach, defrosted
and undrained

1 teaspoon Worcestershire sauce

¼ teaspoon salt

¼ teaspoon pepper

1 tablespoon butter

1 tablespoon flour

Bring the milk and broth to a boil in a large pot. Stir in the spinach,
Worcestershire sauce, salt, and pepper. Bring the mixture to a second boil,
lower the heat, and simmer the soup, partially covered, for 15 minutes.

While the soup is simmering, melt the butter in a small pan over medium
heat, add the flour and cook, stirring constantly, until the roux is golden
brown. Add 1 cup of the soup to the roux and whisk to combine. Return the
mixture to the soup pot. Blend well and heat the soup for 5 more minutes.

Serve hot.

Nutritional Analysis

Per Serving

Calories (kcal)	107.5	Cholesterol (mg)	8.0
Total Fat (g)	3.2	Dietary Fiber (g)	4.6
Saturated Fat (g)	1.8	% Calories from Fat	19.9
Monounsaturated Fat (g)	0.8	Vitamin C (mg)	39.0
Polyunsaturated Fat (g)	0.3	Vitamin A (i.u.)	12,005.0

Tomato Soup with Parmesan Cheese

*This is a delicious and easy way to use an abundance of fresh tomatoes,
and a healthy way as well, with each portion containing 160 percent
of the recommended daily allowance of beta-carotene
and 66 percent of the RDA of vitamin C.*

Makes 8 servings

10 large tomatoes

1 tablespoon butter

3 medium carrots, unpeeled, scrubbed, and minced

1 stalk celery, minced

2 medium yellow onions, minced

½ teaspoon sugar

½ teaspoon chopped fresh basil

½ teaspoon dried thyme

½ teaspoon salt

¼ teaspoon pepper

4 tablespoons fresh grated Parmesan cheese

4 tablespoons chopped fresh parsley

Peel, seed, and chop the tomatoes (See Index.).

Heat the butter in a large pot over medium-low heat. Add the carrot, celery, and onion and sauté the vegetables for 20 minutes, or until they're soft (don't allow the vegetables to brown). Add the tomato, sugar, basil, thyme, salt, and pepper to the pot and cook the mixture for 30 minutes. (The soup may be pureed at this point, if a smooth consistency is desired, or it may be left with its texture.)

Serve the soup hot, garnishing each serving with 1½ teaspoons of the Parmesan and 1½ teaspoons of the parsley.

Nutritional Analysis

Per Serving

Calories (kcal)	92.7	Cholesterol (mg)	5.0
Total Fat (g)	2.4	Dietary Fiber (g)	3.0
Saturated Fat (g)	1.3	% Calories from Fat	21.0
Monounsaturated Fat (g)	0.6	Vitamin C (mg)	40.0
Polyunsaturated Fat (g)	0.2	Vitamin A (i.u.)	7,980.0

Salads

3

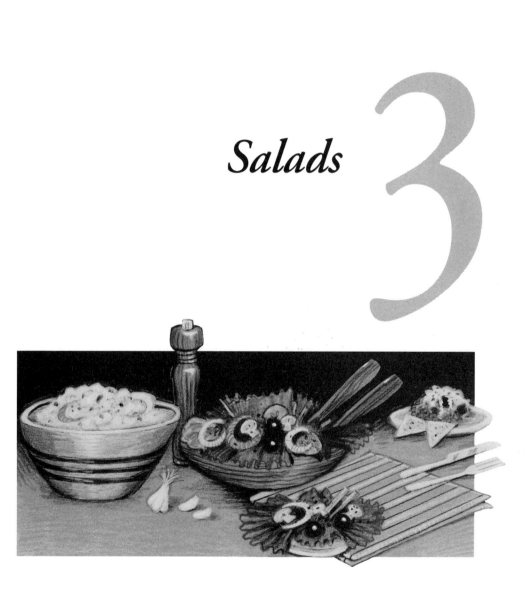

A well-planned salad can be the perfect course. It is quick and simple to prepare, contains varied textures and tastes, looks fresh and appealing, and—most important—fills many requirements of a cancer risk-reduction eating plan. The best salads are high in beta-carotene and vitamin C and low in fat, and contain a substantial amount of dietary fiber. Make delicious and nutritious combinations from fresh leafy greens; cruciferous vegetables; fruits rich in vitamin C; vegetables high in beta-carotene; high-fiber legumes, grains (which are a good source of vitamin E), and beans; and lean meats, fish, and poultry.

Salads are not just for dinner! Begin breakfast or brunch with fresh fruit compote instead of a glass of juice. If you use fruits such as apples, peaches, or nectarines in the salad, sprinkle them with a little fresh lemon juice to prevent discoloration (which happens almost immediately). For the maximum intake of vitamins and fiber, leave the skin on all soft fruits whenever possible. And when using grapefruit and oranges, use the whole fruit—vitamins and fiber are not only in the flesh of the fruit itself but also in the white skin and the translucent membranes separating the sections. The amounts may be minimal, but they add up. Whenever possible, use every part of fruits and vegetables in food preparation.

Eat a fresh vegetable or leafy green salad of your creation at both lunch and dinner. For something a little unusual, try Mustard Greens with Mango-Lime Vinaigrette, Carrots in Fresh Basil Vinaigrette, or Spinach Salad with Orange and Sweet Potato Garnish.

Since "salad" means "lettuce" to many people, remember this basic rule when preparing salads: the darker and more colorful the lettuce leaf, the more vitamins it contains. Experiment with chicory, escarole, tangy and pungent mustard greens, spinach, watercress, and carrot tops. To add vitamins to a pale Belgian endive or iceberg lettuce salad, mix the greens with a darker lettuce such as watercress and add a ripe tomato (otherwise, you are basically eating dressing).

Never soak lettuce; you will lose some of the water-soluble vitamins to the water. Just rinse leafy greens with cool water and pat them dry or spin them dry in a salad spinner. Store whole leaves in the refrigerator in an airtight plastic bag or other container. When you are ready to serve the salad, tear or cut the greens into bite-size pieces. Then add other fruits or vegetables such as tomatoes, carrots, or peppers, cutting them up at the last minute so they won't wilt or dry out.

A salad of crisp greens, fresh vegetables, and a good dressing is a fine addition to any meal, but don't stop there: raid your refrigerator and pantry for hearty, healthful extras. Cold brown rice with its crunchy texture is delicious in a salad and also adds vitamins and fiber. The same is true for garbanzos, peas, lima beans, and kidney beans. These legumes are chewy and satisfying, fill you up, and are low in fat, especially compared with a serving of meat. And just a ½ cup cooked portion will add 5 to 10 grams of fiber to your meal. (To store canned kidney beans, rinse them thoroughly after opening. Otherwise the thick packing liquid becomes rancid within a couple of days.)

This chapter offers some interesting and flavorful dishes. Try Asian Sesame Potato Salad in the winter months when many fresh vegetables are expensive; Sesame Orange Noodle Salad at a buffet supper; or Roasted Fennel and Pear Salad with Balsamic-Pear Dressing when the entree calls for a salad with a touch of sweetness.

Summer is the perfect time for salad. No meal could be more satisfying on a steamy summer night than Papaya and Cucumber Salad. Or for a light lunch on the patio, serve Lentil Salad with Feta Cheese or Shredded Chicken Salad. Calorie counters will appreciate Sweet-and-Sour Red Cabbage, Carrots in Fresh Basil Vinaigrette, and Zesty Lemon Broccoli among others in this chapter.

Any salad is incomplete without the right dressing. Chapter 8, "Sauces, Salad Dressings, and Condiments," suggests many delicious dressings, from piquant spicy Ginger-Soy Dressing to delicate Asian Raspberry Vinegar Dressing.

Your gorgeous salads will be sought out for picnics and all kinds of parties. And who will ever guess that your delicious salads also provide such a wealth of healthful food!

Asian Sesame Potato Salad

This recipe makes wonderful warm potato salad as well as being delicious chilled.
To serve the salad warm, heat the dressing and toss it with warm potatoes.
It is satisfying and contains a good amount of dietary fiber.

Makes 6 servings

2 tablespoons sesame oil (Asian variety)

3 tablespoons low-sodium soy sauce

3 tablespoons rice wine vinegar

¼ cup water

¼ teaspoon dry mustard

¼ teaspoon white pepper

2½ pounds red potatoes, unpeeled

2 teaspoons sesame seeds

2 stalks celery, sliced diagonally

2 scallions, sliced diagonally

1 8-ounce can sliced water chestnuts

To make the dressing, whisk together the oil, soy sauce, vinegar, water, mustard, and white pepper. Set the mixture aside to allow the flavors to develop.

Quarter the potatoes; boil them until tender, about 15 minutes.

While the potatoes are cooking, toast the sesame seeds in a dry frying pan over medium-low heat for 5 minutes (shaking the pan often to prevent burning), or until they begin to crackle and turn a golden brown color. Allow the seeds to cool for a few minutes.

Drain the potatoes and allow them to cool briefly. When the potatoes are cool enough to handle (but still warm), cut the quarters into cubes and toss them with the dressing in a large bowl. Add the celery, scallion, and water chestnuts and toss to combine them with the dressing and potatoes.

Sprinkle the toasted sesame seeds over the salad before serving.

Nutritional Analysis

Per Serving

Calories (kcal)	200.6	Cholesterol (mg)	0.0
Total Fat (g)	5.3	Dietary Fiber (g)	3.8
Saturated Fat (g)	0.8	% Calories from Fat	22.8
Monounsaturated Fat (g)	2.0	Vitamin C (mg)	38.0
Polyunsaturated Fat (g)	2.2	Vitamin A (i.u.)	204.0

BABY GREENS WITH ROQUEFORT, ALMONDS, AND APPLES

The rich Roquefort cheese and crunchy sliced almonds give this salad a rich taste, yet it is low in fat and has a significant amount of beta-carotene and dietary fiber. Bagel croutons add interest and have a wonderful texture.

Makes 8 servings

2 medium red apples, sliced

4 tablespoons fresh lemon juice

2 bagels

¼ cup sliced almonds

3 tablespoons rice wine vinegar

3 tablespoons low-fat chicken broth

1 teaspoon sugar

½ teaspoon salt

¼ teaspoon white pepper

10 cups baby lettuce leaves

2 ounces crumbled Roquefort cheese

Preheat the oven to 350°F.

Toss the apple slices with 1 tablespoon of the lemon juice to prevent them from darkening and set them aside.

Cut the bagels into ½-inch slices with a serrated knife. Place the slices on a baking sheet and toast them for 15 minutes, or until they're crisp and golden.

Meanwhile, toast the almonds in a dry frying pan over medium-low heat for 3 to 5 minutes (shaking the pan often to prevent burning), or until they're golden brown.

Make the dressing by whisking together the vinegar, the remaining 3 tablespoons lemon juice, the broth, sugar, salt, and white pepper. In a large bowl, toss the lettuce with the dressing.

Arrange the salad on a platter and sprinkle the apple slices, bagel "croutons," almonds, and Roquefort cheese on top.

Nutritional Analysis

Per Serving

Calories (kcal)	163.1	Cholesterol (mg)	5.0
Total Fat (g)	5.6	Dietary Fiber (g)	4.7
Saturated Fat (g)	1.6	% Calories from Fat	28.1
Monounsaturated Fat (g)	2.1	Vitamin C (mg)	29.0
Polyunsaturated Fat (g)	1.1	Vitamin A (i.u.)	2,937.0

CARROTS IN FRESH BASIL VINAIGRETTE

This dish could also be the hot vegetable course. It serves six people using only 1 tablespoon of oil in total. This recipe wins the prize for the most beta-carotene in the whole book.

Makes 6 servings

1½ pounds carrots, unpeeled, scrubbed, and sliced

1 tablespoon olive oil

2 tablespoons white wine vinegar

3 tablespoons low-fat chicken broth

2 teaspoons sugar

½ teaspoon salt

¼ teaspoon pepper

3 tablespoons chopped fresh basil

3 tablespoons chopped fresh parsley

Steam the carrots just until they're fork-tender, and drain them (save the liquid to add to soup). Combine all the remaining ingredients to make the dressing and toss it with the carrot slices while they are still warm.

Serve the salad at room temperature or slightly chilled.

Nutritional Analysis

Per Serving

Calories (kcal)	71.1	Cholesterol (mg)	0.0
Total Fat (g)	2.5	Dietary Fiber (g)	3.1
Saturated Fat (g)	0.3	% Calories from Fat	28.7
Monounsaturated Fat (g)	1.7	Vitamin C (mg)	12.0
Polyunsaturated Fat (g)	0.3	Vitamin A (i.u.)	28,545.0

French Potato Salad

A tangy twist on the usual mayonnaise-laden potato salad
(with lots of beta-carotene and vitamin C as well).

Makes 8 servings

8 medium red potatoes

2 medium carrots, peeled and grated

¾ cup chopped green bell pepper

¾ cup chopped red onion

2 tablespoons olive oil

5 tablespoons low-sodium chicken broth

2 tablespoons white wine vinegar

1 tablespoon fresh lemon juice

1½ teaspoons Dijon mustard

½ teaspoon salt

¼ teaspoon black pepper

Cut the potatoes into bite-size pieces and steam them until they're fork-tender (about 8 minutes). Allow the potato pieces to cool a bit, then toss them in a large bowl with the carrot, bell pepper, and onion. Combine the remaining ingredients to make the dressing. Pour the dressing over the vegetables and gently, but thoroughly, toss the salad.

Serve the salad at room temperature or slightly chilled.

Nutritional Analysis

Per Serving

Calories (kcal)	113.4	Cholesterol (mg)	0.0
Total Fat (g)	3.6	Dietary Fiber (g)	2.3
Saturated Fat (g)	0.5	% Calories from Fat	27.0
Monounsaturated Fat (g)	2.5	Vitamin C (mg)	27.0
Polyunsaturated Fat (g)	0.4	Vitamin A (i.u.)	4,555.0

HOT SPINACH AND WATERCRESS SALAD WITH ENOKI MUSHROOMS

This salad calls for bacon, which may be purchased from the butcher by the slice. As the consumption of bacon is something we do less of, we suggest buying only the amount needed for use in a recipe. If you must purchase a full package, consider freezing what is not needed and saving it for another time when a couple of slices in a recipe will help satisfy an urge for this salty, rich food.

Makes 6 servings

1 orange

2 slices bacon

3 tablespoons balsamic vinegar

¼ teaspoon salt

¼ teaspoon pepper

1 teaspoon sesame seeds

1 pound spinach, washed and trimmed

1 bunch watercress, washed and trimmed

½ cup thinly sliced red onion

3½ ounces enoki mushrooms, trimmed

Peel the orange, leaving some of the vitamin-rich white part, and slice it cross-wise, saving the juice to use in the dressing.

Fry the bacon in a large frying pan until the strips are crisp. Drain the bacon, crumble it, and set it aside.

Add the reserved orange juice and the vinegar, salt, pepper, and sesame seeds to the bacon drippings in the pan. Heat the mixture over medium-high heat and, when it's hot, add the spinach and watercress, tossing just until the greens are slightly wilted. Place the salad mixture on a serving platter or individual plates. Arrange the orange and onion slices, mushrooms, and crumbled bacon on top. Serve immediately.

Nutritional Analysis

Per Serving

Calories (kcal)	46.3	Cholesterol (mg)	2.0
Total Fat (g)	1.6	Dietary Fiber (g)	2.1
Saturated Fat (g)	0.4	% Calories from Fat	26.8
Monounsaturated Fat (g)	0.6	Vitamin C (mg)	29.0
Polyunsaturated Fat (g)	0.3	Vitamin A (i.u.)	3,938.0

Lentil Salad with Feta Cheese

We have revised this recipe from the original book, since it was one of the most popular. Watercress adds a fresh, crunchy texture while the creamy feta imparts a richness that pairs beautifully with the naturally peppery lentils.

Makes 6 servings

1 cup lentils	½ teaspoon dried oregano
2 tablespoons vegetable broth	¼ teaspoon salt
2 tablespoons red wine vinegar	¼ teaspoon pepper
1 tablespoon olive oil	1 cup chopped watercress
2 cloves garlic, minced	2 ounces crumbled feta cheese

Place the lentils in a saucepan and cover them with 3 cups of water. Bring the water to a boil, reduce heat, and let the lentils simmer, covered, for 30 minutes, or until they're tender but not mushy. Drain them well and allow them to cool.

Make the dressing by combining the remaining ingredients except the watercress and feta. At serving time, gently toss the lentils with the dressing, watercress, and cheese.

Nutritional Analysis

Per Serving

Calories (kcal)	159.6	Cholesterol (mg)	8.0
Total Fat (g)	4.7	Dietary Fiber (g)	10.0
Saturated Fat (g)	1.8	% Calories from Fat	25.5
Monounsaturated Fat (g)	2.2	Vitamin C (mg)	5.0
Polyunsaturated Fat (g)	0.4	Vitamin A (i.u.)	397.0

Mustard Greens
with Mango-Lime Vinaigrette

We developed this recipe using Japanese mustard greens (imisuna) that are grown by farmers in Sonoma County, California. Any mustard greens may be used, but choose bunches with smaller leaves, if possible, as they will be more tender than the larger ones. This salad contains high levels of beta-carotene and vitamin C.

Makes 6 servings

12 cups mustard greens (about 1 pound)

½ cup fresh mango chunks

3 tablespoons fresh orange juice

1 tablespoon olive oil

1 tablespoon mild balsamic vinegar

2 tablespoons fresh lime juice

½ teaspoon curry powder

½ teaspoon sugar

¼ teaspoon salt

⅛ teaspoon white pepper

⅔ cup cooked brown rice

Wash the greens, remove the tough lower stems, and tear the leaves in bite-size pieces. Place them in a large salad bowl.

To make the dressing, combine the remaining ingredients, except the rice, in a food processor and blend until they're well mixed.

Just before serving, gently but thoroughly toss the greens with the dressing. Sprinkle the greens with the cooked rice and serve.

Nutritional Analysis

Per Serving

Calories (kcal)	84.3	Cholesterol (mg)	0.0
Total Fat (g)	2.7	Dietary Fiber (g)	2.7
Saturated Fat (g)	0.4	% Calories from Fat	26.3
Monounsaturated Fat (g)	1.8	Vitamin C (mg)	81.0
Polyunsaturated Fat (g)	0.3	Vitamin A (i.u.)	5,893.0

Papaya and Cucumber Salad

Papayas, so delicate and delicious, used to be unavailable in most states except for Hawaii and California. This fruit, rich in vitamin C and beta-carotene, is now sold everywhere.

Makes 6 servings

2 medium papayas

1 medium cucumber

6 cups romaine lettuce (about 6 ounces)

1 tablespoon vegetable oil

3 tablespoons white wine vinegar

1 tablespoon sugar

3 tablespoons fresh orange juice

½ teaspoon minced onion

⅓ teaspoon Dijon mustard

¼ teaspoon salt

Peel the papayas and slice them into bite-size pieces (reserve 2 teaspoons of the seeds for the dressing). Peel the cucumber, if desired, and slice it. Wash and dry the lettuce and tear it into bite-size pieces. Chill the lettuce until serving time.

To make the dressing, place the remaining ingredients, including the papaya seeds, in a blender and process the mixture until well blended—the papaya seeds should look like specks of pepper.

At serving time, toss the papaya, cucumber, and lettuce in a salad bowl with the dressing.

Nutritional Analysis

Per Serving

Calories (kcal)	80.5	Cholesterol (mg)	0.0
Total Fat (g)	2.6	Dietary Fiber (g)	2.9
Saturated Fat (g)	0.3	% Calories from Fat	27.1
Monounsaturated Fat (g)	1.4	Vitamin C (mg)	64.0
Polyunsaturated Fat (g)	0.6	Vitamin A (i.u.)	1,788.0

Pear and Endive Salad with Warm Citrus Dressing

This endive and pear salad is perfect for fall or winter. It is sophisticated, with the accents of lime juice, and is simple to make. Your guests will never believe it's low in fat because it's so delicious.

Makes 6 servings

1 medium onion bagel

2 cups unpeeled pear cubes

2½ tablespoons fresh orange juice

3 heads Belgian endive, sliced into ¼-inch pieces

1 tablespoon sugar

4 teaspoons canola oil

1 tablespoon fresh lime juice

¼ teaspoon salt

⅛ teaspoon white pepper

Preheat the oven to 350°F.

Cut the bagel into ½-inch cubes, using a serrated knife. Place the cubes on a baking sheet, and bake them for 15 minutes, or until crisp.

Combine the pear, 1 tablespoon of the orange juice, and the endive in a large bowl and set it aside.

To make the dressing, combine the remaining 1½ tablespoons orange juice, the sugar, oil, lime juice, salt, and white pepper in a small saucepan and cook the mixture over medium heat for 3 minutes, or until the sugar melts—*do not boil.*

Immediately pour the dressing over the pear mixture, tossing gently to coat the fruit. Top with the bagel croutons and serve immediately.

Nutritional Analysis

Per Serving

Calories (kcal)	145.1	Cholesterol (mg)	1.0
Total Fat (g)	3.9	Dietary Fiber (g)	7.3
Saturated Fat (g)	0.5	% Calories from Fat	22.4
Monounsaturated Fat (g)	1.9	Vitamin C (mg)	21.0
Polyunsaturated Fat (g)	1.0	Vitamin A (i.u.)	4,538.0

Potato Salad

A traditional version of potato salad is about 68 percent calories from fat. This one is only 28.4 percent calories from fat because chicken broth provides the moisture and there is just enough mayonnaise to give the usual flavor and texture.

Makes 6 servings

1½ pounds potatoes, peeled and cubed

½ cup low-fat chicken broth

1½ tablespoons cider vinegar

¾ cup chopped yellow onion

¾ cup chopped celery

¼ cup chopped dill pickle

3 tablespoons finely chopped fresh parsley

½ teaspoon salt

½ teaspoon white pepper

2 hard-cooked chopped egg whites

2 tablespoons mayonnaise

Boil the potatoes just until tender. Drain them well and toss them gently with the broth, vinegar, onion, celery, pickle, parsley, salt, and white pepper. Marinate the mixture for 10 minutes, tossing gently once or twice.

Add the egg whites and mayonnaise and toss to combine.

Nutritional Analysis

Per Serving

Calories (kcal)	120.6	Cholesterol (mg)	2.0
Total Fat (g)	4.1	Dietary Fiber (g)	2.2
Saturated Fat (g)	0.6	% Calories from Fat	28.4
Monounsaturated Fat (g)	1.1	Vitamin C (mg)	22.0
Polyunsaturated Fat (g)	2.0	Vitamin A (i.u.)	334.0

Roasted Fennel and Pear Salad with Balsamic-Pear Dressing

Roasting tones down the sharpness of the fennel and enhances the sweetness of the pears in this salad. The roasted pears also produce a wonderfully unusual dressing. This dish is both low in fat and rich in beta-carotene.

Makes 4 servings

2 medium firm, ripe pears
8 ounces fennel bulbs
  (1 medium)
2 teaspoons olive oil
⅓ cup low-fat chicken broth

2 tablespoons balsamic vinegar
¼ teaspoon salt
¼ teaspoon white pepper
6 cups mixed salad greens
  (packed)

Preheat the oven to 400°F.

Halve and core the pears and place the sections, cut-side up, in a baking dish with sides. Core and quarter the fennel bulb(s) and place the pieces in the dish with the pears. Combine the oil and broth and drizzle the mixture over the pears and fennel. Roast the pears and fennel for 10 minutes, then turn each piece over and roast the other sides for 5 more minutes, just until the pears are tender. Remove the pears, and roast the fennel for 15 minutes more. Transfer the fennel to a plate with the pears, reserving any cooking liquid.

Thinly slice the fennel and two of the pear halves lengthwise and let them cool completely. Peel the remaining two pear halves and place them in a food processor. Add the reserved cooking liquid, vinegar, salt, and white pepper and blend until the mixture is very smooth.

Place the greens on a serving platter or four individual plates. Arrange the fennel and pear slices over the greens and drizzle the dressing on top.

Nutritional Analysis

Per Serving

Calories (kcal)	114.8	Cholesterol (mg)	0.0
Total Fat (g)	2.9	Dietary Fiber (g)	4.1
Saturated Fat (g)	0.3	% Calories from Fat	20.2
Monounsaturated Fat (g)	1.7	Vitamin C (mg)	23.0
Polyunsaturated Fat (g)	0.4	Vitamin A (i.u.)	2,390.0

Sesame Orange Noodle Salad

Leftover meat or chicken could be added to make this a main-dish salad.
It can also be served as a hot pasta dish, if desired.

Makes 6 servings

12 ounces spaghetti

3 medium carrots, grated

¾ cup sliced scallion (about 6)

⅓ cup chopped fresh cilantro

2 tablespoons sesame oil (Asian variety)

¼ cup soy sauce

¼ cup rice wine vinegar

¼ cup low-fat chicken broth

2 tablespoons grated orange peel

1 tablespoon sugar

Cook the spaghetti according to the package directions until tender, drain it, and toss it with the carrot, scallion, and cilantro. Make the dressing by combining the remaining ingredients.

Toss the dressing well with the spaghetti and vegetables.

Nutritional Analysis

Per Serving

Calories (kcal)	286.9	Cholesterol (mg)	0.0
Total Fat (g)	5.5	Dietary Fiber (g)	2.8
Saturated Fat (g)	0.8	% Calories from Fat	17.2
Monounsaturated Fat (g)	1.9	Vitamin C (mg)	11.0
Polyunsaturated Fat (g)	2.3	Vitamin A (i.u.)	9,091.0

SHREDDED CHICKEN SALAD

This type of salad is usually very high in fat. But instead of flouring and deep-frying the chicken, we use brown rice for extra texture and flavor. While the salad contains enough sesame oil to give the traditional flavor, chicken broth is used as the base of the dressing instead of vegetable or peanut oil.

Makes 8 servings

2 tablespoons soy sauce

2 tablespoons sherry

16 ounces cooked and shredded chicken breast

4 scallions

1 pound Chinese cabbage, shredded

2 cups cooked brown rice

1 ounce chopped dry-roasted cashews

½ cup chopped fresh cilantro

1 8-ounce can sliced water chestnuts, drained

½ cup low-fat chicken broth

1 tablespoon sesame oil (Asian variety)

¼ teaspoon dry mustard

Combine the soy sauce and sherry and marinate the shredded chicken in the mixture for 30 minutes.

Slice the scallions lengthwise, at an angle. Place the shredded cabbage in a large serving bowl and top it with the chicken, scallion, rice, cashews, cilantro, and water chestnuts. Combine the remaining ingredients to make the dressing and pour it over the salad. Toss well to coat the pieces evenly and serve.

Nutritional Analysis

Per Serving

Calories (kcal)	233.4	Cholesterol (mg)	39.0
Total Fat (g)	7.6	Dietary Fiber (g)	3.5
Saturated Fat (g)	1.7	% Calories from Fat	28.9
Monounsaturated Fat (g)	3.2	Vitamin C (mg)	63.0
Polyunsaturated Fat (g)	2.0	Vitamin A (i.u.)	1,846.0

SPINACH SALAD WITH ORANGE AND SWEET POTATO GARNISH

This colorful salad has a variety of flavors, including sweet and piquant. The vitamin content is very high. This dish offers so much for a simply prepared course in terms of taste, nutrients, and fiber. Add some cooked seafood or chicken, and you have a wonderful light meal.

Makes 6 servings

2 8-ounce sweet potatoes

2 large oranges

3 tablespoons fresh orange juice

1½ tablespoons olive oil

2 tablespoons fresh lime juice

4 teaspoons sugar

¼ teaspoon salt

¼ teaspoon white pepper

1 pound fresh spinach, stemmed and torn

Pierce the sweet potatoes, then bake them in a 425°F oven for 45 minutes, or until tender, or in a microwave for about 5 minutes. Slice the potatoes. Peel off the outer layer of the oranges with a knife, leaving some of the white pith (it contains many of the vitamins), then slice the oranges.

To make the dressing, whisk together the orange juice, oil, lime juice, sugar, salt, and white pepper.

Place the spinach on a platter or on individual plates. Arrange the orange and sweet potato slices on top of the spinach and drizzle the dressing over them.

Nutritional Analysis

Per Serving

Calories (kcal)	107.8	Cholesterol (mg)	0.0
Total Fat (g)	3.8	Dietary Fiber (g)	3.6
Saturated Fat (g)	0.5	% Calories from Fat	29.1
Monounsaturated Fat (g)	2.5	Vitamin C (mg)	47.0
Polyunsaturated Fat (g)	0.4	Vitamin A (i.u.)	6,735.0

Sweet-and-Sour Red Cabbage Salad

It takes only minutes to prepare this hot, slightly crunchy salad. Beyond the quick preparation, the beauty of this dish lies in its colorful and delicious pairing with poultry, pork, or our own Spicy Italian Sausages.

Makes 4 servings

2 cups coarsely shredded red cabbage

3 tablespoons sugar

½ teaspoon salt

¼ cup water

2 tablespoons vinegar

1 teaspoon butter

1 medium Granny Smith apple, unpeeled and sliced

Combine all the ingredients, except the apple, in a medium saucepan; toss well. Cover the pan and cook over medium-low heat for about 8 minutes, or until the cabbage is crisp-tender. Add the apple slices; cover and cook for 5 minutes. Remove the cover and cook for 10 minutes longer, or until liquid has almost evaporated, stirring occasionally.

Nutritional Analysis

Per Serving

Calories (kcal)	68.7	Cholesterol (mg)	3.0
Total Fat (g)	1.1	Dietary Fiber (g)	1.2
Saturated Fat (g)	0.6	% Calories from Fat	12.9
Monounsaturated Fat (g)	0.3	Vitamin C (mg)	17.0
Polyunsaturated Fat (g)	0.1	Vitamin A (i.u.)	47.0

Taco Salad

This salad has such a variety of flavor and texture, plus moisture from the beans and tomatoes, that we find it to be delicious without adding dressing.

Makes 6 servings

3 corn tortillas

1 pound ground turkey

3 cups canned kidney beans, drained

1 teaspoon chili powder

1 large head iceberg lettuce

4 scallions, sliced

6 tomatoes, chopped

3 ounces grated mozzarella cheese, part skim

1½ cups chopped green bell pepper

With the tortillas, prepare Baked Tortilla Chips (See Index.).

In a nonstick pan, cook the ground turkey until it's crumbly and cooked through. Add the kidney beans and chili powder and cook 5 minutes longer.

Place the lettuce, scallion, tomato, cheese, and bell pepper in a large salad bowl. Add the turkey mixture and toss well. Break up the baked tortilla chips and scatter them over the top.

Toss the salad and serve immediately.

Nutritional Analysis

Per Serving

Calories (kcal)	368.2	Cholesterol (mg)	67.0
Total Fat (g)	10.1	Dietary Fiber (g)	6.4
Saturated Fat (g)	3.4	% Calories from Fat	23.7
Monounsaturated Fat (g)	3.2	Vitamin C (mg)	93.0
Polyunsaturated Fat (g)	2.2	Vitamin A (i.u.)	1,902.0

Warm Blue Cheese and Pear Slaw

Although cabbage is thought of as a humble food, combining it with balsamic vinegar, fresh pear, and blue cheese elevates this cancer-fighting cruciferous vegetable. This dish is a treat in terms of taste and texture.

Makes 4 servings

¼ cup water

1 tablespoon sugar

1 tablespoon balsamic vinegar

½ teaspoon salt

¼ teaspoon white pepper

2 cups finely shredded red cabbage

1 pear, unpeeled and cubed

2 tablespoons crumbled blue cheese

Bring the water, sugar, vinegar, salt, and white pepper to a boil in a large pot or frying pan. Cover the pan, reduce the heat, and simmer the mixture for 1 minute. Add the cabbage and sauté for 2 minutes. Add the pear and sauté for 1 minute.

Transfer the slaw to a serving platter or plates and sprinkle the crumbled blue cheese on top. Serve immediately.

Nutritional Analysis

Per Serving

Calories (kcal)	67.8	Cholesterol (mg)	3.0
Total Fat (g)	1.5	Dietary Fiber (g)	1.9
Saturated Fat (g)	0.8	% Calories from Fat	18.3
Monounsaturated Fat (g)	0.4	Vitamin C (mg)	18.0
Polyunsaturated Fat (g)	0.1	Vitamin A (i.u.)	53.0

WILTED CAESAR SALAD

This is not the texture of your ordinary Caesar salad with the dressing thickly coating each piece of lettuce. Ours has all the pungent garlicky taste of the well-known salad, but is much lower in fat.

Makes 6 servings

2 slices French bread

8 cups torn and packed
romaine lettuce leaves

1 cup sliced fresh mushrooms

¼ cup water

2 tablespoons grated Romano
or Asiago cheese

2 tablespoons red wine vinegar

1½ teaspoons sugar

1 teaspoon anchovy paste

¼ teaspoon pepper

2 cloves garlic, minced

Preheat the oven to 350°F.

Slice the bread into crouton-size pieces, place them on a baking sheet, and toast them for 5 minutes, or until crisp. Place the lettuce and mushrooms in a large bowl and set it aside.

Make the dressing by combining the remaining ingredients in a blender and processing until smooth. Pour the dressing into a small saucepan and bring it to a boil. Immediately pour the dressing over the lettuce and mushrooms and toss gently.

Serve topped with the French bread croutons.

Nutritional Analysis

Per Serving

Calories (kcal)	55.4	Cholesterol (mg)	2.0
Total Fat (g)	1.2	Dietary Fiber (g)	2.2
Saturated Fat (g)	0.5	% Calories from Fat	18.8
Monounsaturated Fat (g)	0.3	Vitamin C (mg)	19.0
Polyunsaturated Fat (g)	0.2	Vitamin A (i.u.)	1,980.0

Zesty Lemon Broccoli

*Broccoli is one of the best anticancer vegetables because it has
high levels of beta-carotene, vitamin C, and dietary fiber.
This is our version of a Florentine dish.*

Makes 6 servings

2 pounds broccoli

3 tablespoons low-fat chicken
   broth

3 tablespoons fresh lemon juice

1½ tablespoons olive oil

1 teaspoon lemon zest

3 cloves garlic, minced

½ teaspoon salt

½ teaspoon white pepper

Separate the broccoli into florets. Peel the stems with a paring knife and slice
them crosswise. Steam the broccoli for about 5 minutes, just until fork-tender.
Remove the broccoli (save the steaming liquid for soup), then quickly immerse
it in very cold water to stop the cooking process. When the broccoli is no
longer hot, drain it.

Make the dressing by combining the remaining ingredients in a blender. Toss
the broccoli with the dressing and let it marinate for a few hours.

Serve at room temperature or slightly chilled.

Nutritional Analysis

Per Serving

Calories (kcal)	82.8	Cholesterol (mg)	0.0
Total Fat (g)	3.0	Dietary Fiber (g)	5.8
Saturated Fat (g)	0.4	% Calories from Fat	27.4
Monounsaturated Fat (g)	1.7	Vitamin C (mg)	181.0
Polyunsaturated Fat (g)	0.6	Vitamin A (i.u.)	3,051.0

Seafood, Poultry, and Meat Entrees

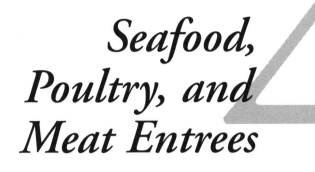

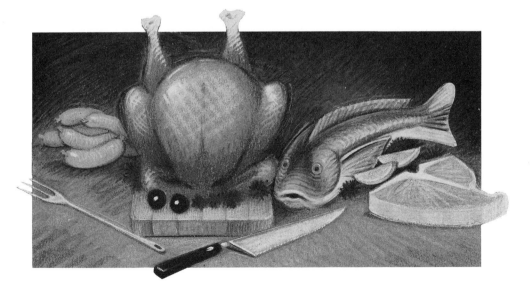

When it's time to prepare the main course, there are many types of seafood, poultry, and meat from which to choose on a cancer risk-reduction eating plan. The focus in this chapter is to keep fat to a minimum, and flavor and creativity to a maximum. Featuring such favorites as shrimp, chicken breasts, scallops, white meat of turkey, sirloin and other lean cuts of beef, veal, lamb, pork tenderloin, and some wonderfully light fish, these dishes will appeal to a wide variety of appetites.

The entrees are designed so that one serving is approximately 3 to 4 ounces of meat, or 4 ounces of seafood or poultry. (This supplies the average adult female with about 62 percent of her daily protein requirement, and the adult male about 49 percent.) Be sure to adhere to this portion size, because lean meats, seafood, and poultry *still* contain 9 percent to 35 percent calories from fat.

Use the following guidelines to plan your menus:

- Eat most often: white meat of turkey (with skin removed), white fish (halibut, flounder, sole, perch, shark, swordfish), water-packed tuna or salmon, chicken breasts (with fat pockets and skin removed), and shellfish such as clams or mussels, lobster, and shrimp, if you are not on a cholesterol-restricted diet.

- Eat in moderation: lean sirloin of beef, ground round steak, dark meat of chicken and turkey, pink or red salmon (fresh or frozen), flank steak, lean cuts of lamb, lean cuts of veal (steaks and chops), and pork tenderloin.

- Eat only occasionally: beef roasts, pork roasts, veal roasts, and lamb chops.

It is worth the time to find a good butcher who will help you select the best lean cuts of meat and then also trim the visible fat. The latter service alone will save you a good amount of preparation time. Then use the cooking methods described in this chapter to ensure tenderness. One basic cooking rule for all meat, seafood, and poultry: never overcook. Besides giving food a tough, hard texture, overcooking ruins the taste.

Seafood

COOKING METHODS

The most popular methods of cooking fish are poaching, broiling, and sautéing because of the delicate texture of the flesh. These methods take only a few minutes until the fish becomes opaque.

Sauté fish in a scant amount of oil, butter, or margarine. Or better yet (if you are watching cholesterol), use a nonfat cooking spray in a treated pan.

Poach firm-fleshed fish in simmering liquid (wine, juices, or broth) for about 8 to 10 minutes, or until the fish becomes opaque.

You can also bake fish wrapped in foil or lettuce leaves, or placed in a lightly oiled dish with a small amount of liquid. These methods of baking all ensure that the fish will not dry out. To bake any fish, preheat the oven to 400°F to 450°F. Allow 10 minutes of cooking time per inch of thickness of the fish. If you are going to stuff the fish, as in Fillet of Sole with Stuffing, measure the thickness after it has been stuffed.

A light and luscious entree is Orange Roughy in Cilantro-Lime Sauce. It has only 108 calories per serving and is quick to prepare. To avoid that occasional "fishy" smell in the house, soak fresh or frozen fish fillets in milk for 8 to 12 hours in the refrigerator.

CRAB CAKES

This recipe, adapted from a Cajun favorite, is 65 percent lower in fat than most crab cake recipes. Serve the cakes with Mustard Greens with Mango-Lime Vinaigrette from our "Salads" chapter.

Makes 6 servings

1 tablespoon butter

¼ cup finely chopped green onion

¼ cup finely chopped fresh parsley

6 ounces crab meat

½ cup dry unseasoned bread crumbs

1 tablespoon Dijon mustard

1 teaspoon Worcestershire sauce

1 clove garlic, minced

⅛ teaspoon hot pepper sauce

⅛ teaspoon white pepper

2 egg whites, beaten to a froth

1 lime, cut into 6 wedges

Melt the butter in a skillet, add the onion and parsley and sauté the vegetables over medium-high heat for 3 minutes, stirring often. Reduce the heat to low and add the remaining ingredients, except the egg whites and lime, and cook about 3 minutes longer, stirring gently to keep the mixture light. Remove the skillet from the heat, allow the contents to cool a bit, then gently fold in the egg whites.

Lightly shape the mixture into six cakes. Spray a nonstick skillet with cooking spray and heat it to medium-high. Sauté the cakes for 5 minutes on each side.

Serve the crab cakes hot, with the fresh lime wedges.

Nutritional Analysis

Per Serving

Calories (kcal)	92.6	Cholesterol (mg)	3.0
Total Fat (g)	3.0	Dietary Fiber (g)	0.7
Saturated Fat (g)	1.4	% Calories from Fat	29.3
Monounsaturated Fat (g)	1.0	Vitamin C (mg)	8.0
Polyunsaturated Fat (g)	0.3	Vitamin A (i.u.)	220.0

Fillet of Sole with Stuffing

Flavorful and filling, this entree has only 9.8 percent calories from fat.

Makes 4 servings

6 ounces stuffing cubes (seasoned bread stuffing)

½ cup white wine (or broth)

1 cup chopped celery

1 cup chopped yellow onion

¾ cup fish broth (or chicken broth)

1 pound sole fillet

½ teaspoon dried thyme

¼ teaspoon pepper

Preheat the oven to 300°F.

Place the stuffing cubes in a large bowl. Heat the wine in a medium skillet, add the celery and onion, and sauté the vegetables in the wine until they're softened (about 5 minutes), then add them to the bowl. Toss the sautéed vegetables and stuffing cubes with the fish broth and place the mixture in a casserole dish. Top with the sole, sprinkle with the thyme and pepper, and cover the dish with a lid or foil.

Bake the casserole for 30 minutes.

Nutritional Analysis

Per Serving

Calories (kcal)	293.1	Cholesterol (mg)	4.0
Total Fat (g)	2.1	Dietary Fiber (g)	1.4
Saturated Fat (g)	1.0	% Calories from Fat	9.8
Monounsaturated Fat (g)	0.7	Vitamin C (mg)	6.0
Polyunsaturated Fat (g)	0.4	Vitamin A (i.u.)	96.0

Fish Stew Provençale

With crusty whole-grain bread to dip in the broth, and a salad on the side, this makes a wonderful meal!

Makes 8 servings

2 teaspoons olive oil

1¼ cups chopped yellow onion

2 cloves garlic, minced

2 medium carrots, chopped fine

1 medium tomato, peeled, seeded, and diced

½ teaspoon dried basil

½ teaspoon dried thyme

3½ cups chicken broth

1 24-ounce can clam juice

1 cup dry white wine

1½ teaspoons grated orange peel

8 clams in the shell

2 pounds halibut or other firm fish

½ cup chopped fresh parsley

4 lemons, halved

To make the herb-wine broth, heat the oil in a large pan. Add the onion, garlic, and carrot and sauté the vegetables until the onion is limp. Stir in the tomato, basil, thyme, broth, clam juice, wine, and orange peel. Cover the pan and let the broth simmer for 30 minutes. The broth may be used immediately but is even better if made a day or two ahead and refrigerated until needed.

To assemble the stew, bring the broth to a boil in a large pot or skillet. Stir in the clams and halibut. Bring the mixture to a second boil, reduce the heat, cover the pot, and allow the stew to simmer over medium heat until the clams have opened (about 5 to 10 minutes).

Ladle the broth into bowls and divide the fish and clams among them. Garnish each serving with the parsley and lemon.

Nutritional Analysis

Per Serving

Calories (kcal)	247.7	Cholesterol (mg)	43.0
Total Fat (g)	5.3	Dietary Fiber (g)	1.4
Saturated Fat (g)	0.9	% Calories from Fat	20.6
Monounsaturated Fat (g)	2.1	Vitamin C (mg)	31.0
Polyunsaturated Fat (g)	1.4	Vitamin A (i.u.)	5,127.0

ORANGE ROUGHY
IN CILANTRO-LIME SAUCE

*A wonderful low-calorie entree. Serve the fish with steamed spinach
or baby carrots.*

Makes 4 servings

1 tablespoon olive oil

2 tablespoons fresh lime juice

2 tablespoons chopped fresh
  cilantro

2 cloves garlic, minced

¼ teaspoon salt

⅛ teaspoon pepper

1 pound orange roughy
  fillets (4)

1 lime, quartered

Combine the oil, lime juice, cilantro, garlic, salt, and pepper. Rub the
marinade into the fish. Place the fillets in a zip-lock plastic bag (or in a single
layer in a shallow dish and cover). Close the bag and refrigerate the fish for
15 to 30 minutes.

Coat a nonstick pan with cooking spray and heat it to medium-hot. Place the
fillets in the pan and cook them for 3 minutes, turn them, and cook the other
side for 2 to 3 minutes longer, or until the flesh is opaque all the way through.

Serve the fish with the lime wedges.

Nutritional Analysis

Per Serving

Calories (kcal)	107.8	Cholesterol (mg)	23.0
Total Fat (g)	3.1	Dietary Fiber (g)	0.2
Saturated Fat (g)	0.4	% Calories from Fat	26.1
Monounsaturated Fat (g)	2.2	Vitamin C (mg)	7.0
Polyunsaturated Fat (g)	0.3	Vitamin A (i.u.)	94.0

SALMON WITH CUCUMBER-YOGURT SAUCE

Yogurt replaces the mayonnaise or sour cream traditionally used for this type of sauce, with a delicious and lighter flavor that complements the rich salmon with a refreshingly light taste.

Makes 6 servings

1 cup nonfat yogurt

½ cup peeled and grated cucumber

2 tablespoons finely chopped shallot

1 tablespoon chopped fresh dill weed

1 medium yellow onion, sliced

2 limes, sliced thin

½ tablespoon olive oil

24 ounces salmon steak (3 8-ounce or 6 4-ounce)

1 teaspoon dried thyme

1 teaspoon dried oregano

1 teaspoon dried rosemary

Mix the yogurt, cucumber, shallot, and dill for the sauce. Cover the mixture and chill it for several hours (or up to 2 days).

Arrange half of the onion slices and half of the lime slices in a baking dish just large enough to hold the fish in a single layer. Rub the oil over both sides of the salmon steaks and place the salmon on top of the onion and lime slices. Sprinkle the remaining herbs over both sides of the steaks. Top with the remaining onion and lime slices. Cover the dish and refrigerate it for 4 to 12 hours.

Preheat the oven to 400°F. Uncover the salmon, and bake the steaks until they're just cooked through, about 15 minutes. If you're using 3 8-ounce steaks, gently cut each along the backbone, separating it into two pieces. Transfer the salmon to plates and spoon the chilled sauce over each serving.

Nutritional Analysis
Per Serving

Calories (kcal)	184.0	Cholesterol (mg)	60.0
Total Fat (g)	5.2	Dietary Fiber (g)	0.7
Saturated Fat (g)	0.8	% Calories from Fat	25.9
Monounsaturated Fat (g)	1.9	Vitamin C (mg)	9.0
Polyunsaturated Fat (g)	1.7	Vitamin A (i.u.)	560.0

SCALLOPS WITH POTATOES AND CAVIAR

This elegant light entree or first course can be completely prepared ahead of time and assembled just before eating. The bed of greens supplies a good amount of vitamin C and beta-carotene.

Makes 4 servings

1¼ pounds red potatoes (12 small)

4 teaspoons olive oil

½ teaspoon salt

½ teaspoon white pepper

2 tablespoons rice wine vinegar

12 ounces quartered bay scallops

3 tablespoons low-fat chicken broth

2 tablespoons fresh lemon juice

1 teaspoon lemon zest

6 cups mixed salad greens

1½ teaspoons caviar

Preheat the oven to 400°F.

Place the potatoes in a baking pan and drizzle 2 teaspoons of the oil over them; shake the pan to distribute the oil evenly. Sprinkle the potatoes with ¼ teaspoon each of the salt and pepper and shake the pan again to coat them. Bake the potatoes for 30 minutes, or until tender. Refrigerate them until serving time.

In a saucepan, bring 2 cups of water and the vinegar to a boil. Add the scallops and simmer the mixture for 1 to 2 minutes, or until the scallops are just opaque inside when pierced with a fork. Refrigerate the scallops until serving time.

Make the dressing by whisking together the broth, lemon juice, lemon zest, and the remaining salt, white pepper, and oil.

At serving time, divide the salad greens among six plates. Arrange the scallops and potatoes on the lettuce and drizzle the dressing over them. Top each serving with ¼ teaspoon of the caviar.

Nutritional Analysis

Per Serving

Calories (kcal)	148.6	Cholesterol (mg)	27.0
Total Fat (g)	3.8	Dietary Fiber (g)	2.2
Saturated Fat (g)	0.5	% Calories from Fat	22.7
Monounsaturated Fat (g)	2.3	Vitamin C (mg)	28.0
Polyunsaturated Fat (g)	0.6	Vitamin A (i.u.)	1,596.0

Seafood Étouffée

This is a typical Cajun recipe. It contains just enough oil to retain the richness of texture and goodness of flavor. You won't feel that you're missing anything with the reduction of oil by ⅓ cup from the standard recipe.

Makes 6 servings

1 tablespoon canola oil

1½ cups chopped yellow onion

⅔ cup chopped green bell pepper

1 cup chopped celery

2 cloves garlic, minced

1½ pounds catfish, cut in large pieces

½ pound small cooked shrimp

½ teaspoon dried thyme

½ teaspoon salt

¼ teaspoon cayenne

¼ teaspoon black pepper

¼ teaspoon dried oregano

2 tablespoons tomato paste

1½ cups fish broth or clam juice

2 scallions, sliced thin

⅓ cup chopped fresh parsley

2 cups cooked rice*

Heat the oil in a large dutch oven over medium heat. Add the onion, bell pepper, celery, and garlic and sauté the vegetables for 10 minutes. Place the catfish and shrimp over the sautéed vegetables and keep on low heat. Combine the spices and herbs with the tomato paste and broth and pour the mixture over the seafood. Bring the contents to a boil, then reduce the heat to low, cover the pot, and simmer the stew for 20 minutes. Add the scallion and parsley and simmer for 5 more minutes.

Serve the hot étouffée over rice.

_____

*Begin cooking the rice following the package directions while the étouffée is simmering.

Nutritional Analysis

Per Serving

Calories (kcal)	316.8	Cholesterol (mg)	144.0
Total Fat (g)	7.9	Dietary Fiber (g)	3.3
Saturated Fat (g)	2.1	% Calories from Fat	23.1
Monounsaturated Fat (g)	2.9	Vitamin C (mg)	44.0
Polyunsaturated Fat (g)	2.0	Vitamin A (i.u.)	815.0

SHRIMP JAMBALAYA

This is a delicious and quick version of traditional jambalaya. Be sure to add the cooked shrimp at the very end, boiling just long enough to heat them without overcooking, or they will be tough. If you're on a cholesterol-restricted diet, substitute "mock crab" for the shrimp.

Makes 4 servings

1 cup rice

2 tablespoons butter

1 cup chopped yellow onion

1 cup chopped green bell
  pepper

3 stalks celery, chopped

3 cups low-fat chicken broth

3 fresh tomatoes, chopped
  coarse

¼ cup chopped fresh parsley

½ teaspoon dried thyme

¼ teaspoon garlic powder

¼ teaspoon salt

¼ teaspoon black pepper

⅛ teaspoon cayenne

1 pound cooked shrimp

Begin cooking the rice according to the package directions. While the rice cooks, melt the butter in a large skillet. Add the onion, bell pepper, and celery and sauté the vegetables for 5 minutes. Add the remaining ingredients, except the shrimp, and bring the contents to a boil. Boil gently for 10 minutes, then add the shrimp and cook for 2 minutes more to heat the shrimp through.

Serve over the cooked rice.

Nutritional Analysis

Per Serving

Calories (kcal)	393.9	Cholesterol (mg)	237.0
Total Fat (g)	7.8	Dietary Fiber (g)	3.5
Saturated Fat (g)	4.0	% Calories from Fat	16.8
Monounsaturated Fat (g)	2.0	Vitamin C (mg)	50.0
Polyunsaturated Fat (g)	1.0	Vitamin A (i.u.)	1,491.0

Swordfish and Noodles
in Ginger-Soy Sauce

*This very contemporary dish is elegant. No one will believe that it is
so very low in fat and calories or that it is simple to prepare.*

Makes 4 servings

1 10-ounce package noodles

1 teaspoon ground coriander

½ teaspoon pepper

¼ teaspoon garlic powder

1 pound swordfish

3 tablespoons low-sodium
soy sauce

3 tablespoons rice wine vinegar

3 tablespoons chopped fresh
cilantro

3 tablespoons chopped scallion

1 teaspoon fresh minced ginger

½ teaspoon sugar

Begin cooking the noodles according to the package directions. While the
noodles are cooking, combine the coriander, pepper, and garlic powder and
sprinkle half the mixture on one side of the swordfish. Heat a nonstick pan
(or any pan sprayed with cooking spray) to medium-hot and place the swordfish, seasoned-side down, in the hot pan. Cook the fish for 5 minutes, then
sprinkle the top with the remaining coriander mixture. Turn the fish over and
cook for an additional 5 minutes.

While the noodles and swordfish are cooking, combine the remaining
ingredients to make the ginger sauce. Drain the noodles and toss them with
the sauce.

Place the noodles on a serving platter and arrange the swordfish on top.

Nutritional Analysis

Per Serving

Calories (kcal)	420.8	Cholesterol (mg)	112.0
Total Fat (g)	7.6	Dietary Fiber (g)	2.2
Saturated Fat (g)	1.9	% Calories from Fat	16.4
Monounsaturated Fat (g)	2.6	Vitamin C (mg)	4.0
Polyunsaturated Fat (g)	1.9	Vitamin A (i.u.)	218.0

THAI HALIBUT
IN LEMONGRASS-SESAME SAUCE

*Lemongrass, a staple spice in Thai cooking, is available in most supermarkets.
If lemongrass is not available, use ⅓ cup chopped scallion
and 1 tablespoon lemon zest.*

Makes 4 servings

1 tablespoon finely chopped
lemongrass (outer leaves
removed)

1½ teaspoons sesame oil

2 tablespoons low-sodium
soy sauce

1 tablespoon rice wine vinegar

4 4-ounce pieces halibut

1 lemon, quartered

Combine the lemongrass, oil, soy sauce, and vinegar. Rub the marinade into
the halibut and place the fish in a zip-lock plastic bag (or in a single layer in a
shallow dish and cover). Refrigerate the fish for 15 to 30 minutes.

Heat a large skillet to medium-hot. Place the halibut in the skillet and cook
for 4 minutes, then turn the pieces over and cook them for 3 to 4 minutes
longer, or until the flesh is opaque all the way through (take care not to
overcook, or the fish will be dry).

Serve the halibut with the lemon wedges.

Nutritional Analysis

Per Serving

Calories (kcal)	119.2	Cholesterol (mg)	27.0
Total Fat (g)	3.7	Dietary Fiber (g)	0.3
Saturated Fat (g)	0.5	% Calories from Fat	27.3
Monounsaturated Fat (g)	1.2	Vitamin C (mg)	22.0
Polyunsaturated Fat (g)	1.4	Vitamin A (i.u.)	140.0

Poultry

COOKING METHODS

Chicken

Whole chicken may be roasted at 350°F for 18 to 20 minutes per pound. Baste the chicken often, and remove the skin before serving. You may also poach chicken pieces to keep in the refrigerator as the base of a quick entree, using any of the sauces in Chapter 8.

Small chickens or game hens may be cut in half and broiled for 15 minutes on each side. Baste the chicken with the broth two or three times. Or thinly slice chicken breasts into scaloppine and sauté them.

Chicken may also be braised, making it incredibly tender. Braising is a combination of browning, stewing, and steaming, rendering a tender, moist dish. Lightly brown one cut-up chicken in a small amount of olive or canola oil, add 1 cup broth, cover the pan, and cook the chicken slowly on the stove top or in the oven at 325°F for 1½ hours. For a wonderful meal, add 3 more cups of chicken broth to the braised chicken. Cut up carrots, parsnips, fennel, and celery, add the vegetables to the broth, and simmer the mixture for 45 minutes. When the vegetables are tender, add 2 cups of cooked brown rice and season to taste. This gives you a thick and hearty soup.

If you cook chicken ahead of time and refrigerate it, just add different sauces at your whim, such as our Greek Yogurt-Dill Sauce or Mexican Green Chili Sauce. If you can't live without fried chicken, traditionally high in fat, try our Spicy Fried Chicken or Special Onion-Fried Mandarin Orange Chicken.

Turkey

The most popular and easy way to cook turkey is to roast it whole. Place the bird breast-side up in a large roasting pan and cook it in a 325°F oven. Cooking on low heat keeps it from drying out. Baste the turkey often with the pan juices. An 8- to 12-pound bird should cook for 3½ to 4 hours; the turkey is done when you pierce the thigh and the juices run clear. Remember to remove the skin before serving.

Turkey may also be cut into pieces and poached, as you would chicken. This is a good way to cook turkey for a party. Turkey meat is so versatile. Chili fans will love Turkey in White Bean Chili with Cilantro Cream. It has an authentic

Tex-Mex flavor and, compared with regular commercial chili, 50 percent less fat. For the busy cook, a quickly prepared entree is our Turkey Scaloppine with Lemon Cream Sauce.

Use the breast meat for sandwiches, or roll warm slices around asparagus or broccoli spears. Add one of our light sauces such as Madeira Sauce or Cranberry-Tangerine Sauce. Use the dark meat for kabobs, add it to stir-fried dishes, or combine it with white meat for chunky turkey salad using Greek Yogurt-Dill Sauce or Creamy Chive Sauce instead of mayonnaise.

CHICKEN GUMBO

"Roux" is a blend of oil and flour in equal parts. It is used as the base of many Southern dishes. To reduce fat we discovered a method of "roasting" the flour by itself. This results in the nutty, deep flavor of the roux, but without any oil.

Makes 6 servings

½ cup flour

7 cups low-fat chicken broth

1 cup chopped yellow onion

¼ cup chopped celery

¼ cup chopped green bell pepper

1 pound boned and skinned chicken breasts, cut in strips

1 teaspoon salt

½ teaspoon black pepper

2 cups rice

½ cup chopped fresh parsley

¾ cup chopped scallion

½ teaspoon filé powder

Cook the flour in a large, heavy pot over medium to medium-high heat for 20 to 30 minutes, whisking constantly, until it reaches a golden brown color (like light brown sugar). This step cannot be rushed. Adjust the heat as necessary between medium and medium-high. If the flour begins to smoke or darken too fast, remove the pan from the heat and return it to a slightly lower setting.

Heat 1 cup of the broth and add it to the flour all at once, incorporating it with a whisk. Then add the remaining 6 cups of broth and bring the mixture to a boil, whisking constantly. Reduce the heat and add the onion, celery, bell pepper, chicken, salt, and black pepper. Return the contents to a boil, then reduce the heat to low and cook for 30 minutes.

While the gumbo is simmering, cook the rice according to package directions.

Add the parsley and scallion to the gumbo and cook, covered, for 5 minutes. Remove the pot from the heat and stir in the filé powder.

Serve the gumbo over the cooked rice in soup bowls.

Nutritional Analysis

Per Serving

Calories (kcal)	384.8		Cholesterol (mg)	44.0
Total Fat (g)	1.6		Dietary Fiber (g)	2.3
Saturated Fat (g)	0.4		% Calories from Fat	3.4
Monounsaturated Fat (g)	2.4		Vitamin C (mg)	19.0
Polyunsaturated Fat (g)	0.4		Vitamin A (i.u.)	358.0

Chicken with Salsa and Rice

Here's a meal the kids will enjoy helping to prepare.
Serve at a sleep-over and let everyone pitch in!

Makes 4 servings

1 cup rice cooked according to
package directions

1 16-ounce package frozen corn
(off the cob)

2 cups salsa (good quality)

1 pound skinless, boneless
chicken, cut into strips

Preheat the oven to 350°F.

Begin cooking the rice according to the package directions. While the rice is cooking, combine the corn and ½ cup of the salsa in a small casserole dish. Cover the dish and bake it for 10 minutes.

Combine the chicken strips and the remaining 1½ cups salsa in a separate casserole dish. Cover the casserole and place it in the oven with the corn. Bake both for 20 minutes longer.

Serve the chicken over the cooked rice with the corn salsa.

Nutritional Analysis

Per Serving

Calories (kcal)	429.3	Cholesterol (mg)	66.0
Total Fat (g)	4.5	Dietary Fiber (g)	4.3
Saturated Fat (g)	0.6	% Calories from Fat	9.0
Monounsaturated Fat (g)	0.7	Vitamin C (mg)	44.0
Polyunsaturated Fat (g)	0.8	Vitamin A (i.u.)	1,500.0

CHINESE FAJITAS

Cross-cultural, or fusion, cooking is a style in which an element from one cuisine is paired with flavoring, wrappings, or cooking procedures from another cuisine. This simple mixing and matching is ideal when the same old recipes need a new twist. It adds zest to everyday cooking, as well as to party foods. There is nothing difficult about fusion cooking once you allow your imagination to run free. Some wonderful dishes—such as these Chinese Fajitas—have been born this way. Try some of your own.

Makes 8 servings

1½ pounds boned and skinned chicken breast halves

½ cup plus 2 tablespoons hoisin sauce

1 tablespoon plus 2 teaspoons rice wine vinegar

3½ teaspoons sesame oil (Asian variety)

2 cloves garlic, minced

1 teaspoon minced ginger

1 cup fresh cilantro leaves plus 2 tablespoons chopped fresh cilantro

2 teaspoons plum sauce

2 tablespoons water

1 cup sliced scallion

½ pound snow peas, halved diagonally

8 slices pita bread

Chicken Filling

Remove any fat from the chicken. Combine the 2 tablespoons hoisin sauce, the 1 tablespoon vinegar, 1½ teaspoons of the sesame oil, and the garlic, ginger, and 1 cup cilantro leaves to make the marinade. Refrigerate the chicken in the marinade for 30 minutes. Broil, grill, or barbecue the chicken for 3 to 4 minutes per side (depending on the thickness), or until tender. Cut the breasts at an angle into thin slices and arrange them on a plate.

Hoisin-Cilantro Sauce

Make the sauce by combining the remaining ½ cup hoisin sauce, the plum sauce, the remaining 2 teaspoons each sesame oil and vinegar, the chopped cilantro, and the water.

Place pita bread on a plate. Open the pita rounds and fill them with the chicken, scallion, and snow peas, then spoon the sauce into the stuffed pita.

Nutritional Analysis

Per Serving

Calories (kcal)	337.8	Cholesterol (mg)	52.0
Total Fat (g)	6.6	Dietary Fiber (g)	2.2
Saturated Fat (g)	1.6	% Calories from Fat	18.0
Monounsaturated Fat (g)	4.8	Vitamin C (mg)	25.0
Polyunsaturated Fat (g)	1.8	Vitamin A (i.u.)	175.0

Soy-Sesame Chicken
with Oriental Vegetables

This is a wonderful combination of flavor, color, and texture—without the last-minute chopping usually associated with Chinese food. It is low in fat and high in beta-carotene.

Makes 6 servings

⅓ cup low-sodium soy sauce

¼ cup chopped fresh cilantro

¼ cup chopped scallion

¼ cup plus 2 tablespoons low-fat chicken broth

2 tablespoons chopped fresh ginger

2 tablespoons rice wine vinegar

4 cloves garlic, minced

2 teaspoons hot chili paste with garlic*

4 teaspoons sesame oil (Asian variety)

1½ pounds boned and skinned chicken breast halves (6)

12 ounces baby carrots, sliced thin

12 ounces jicama, julienned

8 ounces snow peas

1 tablespoon sesame seeds

To make the marinade, combine the soy sauce, cilantro, scallion, the ¼ cup broth, the ginger, vinegar, garlic, hot chili paste, and 1 teaspoon of the sesame oil in a bowl. Pour ½ cup of the marinade into a shallow dish. Add the chicken and turn the pieces to coat them. Cover the dish and refrigerate it at least 2 and up to 4 hours.

Bring a medium-size pot of salted water to a boil. Add the carrot slices and let them simmer for 3 minutes. Add the jicama and snow peas and cook them just until tender, about 2 minutes. Drain the liquid from the pot. Refresh the vegetables with cold water and drain again. (The vegetables can be prepared up to 4 hours ahead: cover the cooked vegetables and chill them until the chicken is cooked.)

Drain the chicken. Heat the remaining tablespoon of oil in a heavy, large skillet over medium-high heat. Add the chicken, smooth-side down, and cook it

---

*Found in the Asian section of the market. Also known as "red chili sauce" or "chili garlic sauce," this condiment looks a bit like a very thick salsa.

for 3 minutes. Turn the chicken pieces over and sprinkle them with the sesame seeds. Continue cooking until the chicken is cooked through, about 3 minutes. Transfer the chicken to plates and keep it warm.

Add the remaining 2 tablespoons of broth and the reserved marinade to the skillet. Add the carrot, jicama, and snow peas and stir until the vegetables are heated through, about 3 minutes.

Top the plates of chicken with the vegetables and drizzle the pan juices over each serving.

Nutritional Analysis

Per Serving

Calorie (kcal)	236.5	Cholesterol (mg)	66.0
Total Fat (g)	5.6	Dietary Fiber (g)	5.2
Saturated Fat (g)	1.0	% Calories from Fat	21.5
Monounsaturated Fat (g)	4.9	Vitamin C (mg)	37.0
Polyunsaturated Fat (g)	2.1	Vitamin A (i.u.)	1,244.0

SPECIAL ONION-FRIED MANDARIN ORANGE CHICKEN

*This onion-browned chicken with a reduced sauce studded
with mandarin oranges seems more like a dish from a fine restaurant
than a quickly prepared recipe that's also good for you!*

Makes 6 servings

¼ cup flour	3 tablespoons butter
1½ teaspoons chopped fresh basil	½ cup finely chopped yellow onion
½ teaspoon salt	1 cup low-fat chicken broth
¼ teaspoon cayenne	1 11-ounce can mandarin oranges, drained (save the juice)
1½ pounds boned and skinned chicken breast halves (6)	

Mix the flour, basil, salt, and cayenne. Lightly but evenly dust the chicken with the flour mixture.

In a large skillet, heat the butter until foamy. Add the onion and sauté it for about 5 minutes, or until the onion is lightly browned. Add the chicken and sauté it for 5 minutes on each side, or until the meat is tender. Remove the chicken from the skillet and cover the meat to keep it warm.

Add the broth and ¼ cup of the juice from the drained mandarin oranges to the skillet. Bring the contents to a rolling boil and boil for 2 minutes. Add the oranges and chicken to the skillet and simmer the mixture 2 minutes longer, or until the chicken is hot.

Nutritional Analysis

Per Serving

Calories (kcal)	219.4	Cholesterol (mg)	81.0
Total Fat (g)	7.2	Dietary Fiber (g)	1.3
Saturated Fat (g)	3.9	% Calories from Fat	29.5
Monounsaturated Fat (g)	5.1	Vitamin C (mg)	14.0
Polyunsaturated Fat (g)	0.6	Vitamin A (i.u.)	654.0

SPICY FRIED CHICKEN

*This recipe is a good example of how to get a deep-fried texture
with a small fraction of the fat needed to deep-fry food.*

Makes 6 servings

1½ pounds boned and skinned
 chicken breast halves (6)

½ cup low-fat (1%) buttermilk

¼ cup Dijon mustard

2 teaspoons lemon pepper

2 teaspoons paprika

1½ teaspoons garlic powder

1 teaspoon dried oregano

1 teaspoon dried thyme

½ teaspoon white pepper

6 cups finely crushed cornflakes

Cut any visible fat off the chicken. Combine the remaining ingredients except
the cornflakes. Place the chicken and the buttermilk mixture, separately, in the
freezer for 10 minutes (chilling both immediately before preparing helps the
coating adhere to the chicken). Preheat the oven to 400°F. Coat a baking sheet
with cooking spray.

Dip the breast pieces into the buttermilk mixture, coating both sides
thoroughly. Then dip the coated chicken in the crushed cornflakes, or shake
them together in a plastic bag, coating each piece very well. Place the chicken
on the baking sheet. Spray the top side of each piece with cooking spray. Bake
the chicken on the lowest shelf of the oven for 15 minutes, then turn the
chicken over and bake for 15 minutes longer.

Nutritional Analysis

Per Serving

Calories (kcal)	238.1	Cholesterol (mg)	67.0
Total Fat (g)	2.3	Dietary Fiber (g)	1.3
Saturated Fat (g)	0.5	% Calories from Fat	8.8
Monounsaturated Fat (g)	3.8	Vitamin C (mg)	14.0
Polyunsaturated Fat (g)	0.5	Vitamin A (i.u.)	1,496.0

SPICY SESAME NOODLES
WITH TURKEY AND SCALLOPS

*This is a fun dish to make, with its creamy peanut sauce coating
soft scallops and turkey, punctuated with crunchy grated carrots
and sesame seeds. It can be prepared ahead
and heated at the last minute.*

Makes 8 servings

¼ cup sesame seeds

½ pound scallops

3 tablespoons rice wine
vinegar

2 tablespoons peanut butter

1½ tablespoons honey

¾ teaspoon Dijon mustard

2½ tablespoons low-sodium
soy sauce

1 teaspoon chili oil (oriental
style)

1 tablespoon sesame oil (Asian
variety)

3 tablespoons low-fat chicken
broth

1½ tablespoons fresh orange
juice

1 pound cooked turkey breast,
cut into bite-size pieces

1 cup grated carrot

12 ounces vermicelli

½ cup chopped scallion

Toast the sesame seeds in a frying pan over medium heat for 5 minutes, or
until they start to pop—stirring or shaking the pan constantly. Set the seeds
aside.

In a medium-size saucepan, bring 4 cups of water to a boil. Add the scallops,
return the water to a boil, then reduce the heat and simmer the scallops for a
few minutes, until they turn opaque. Drain the scallops.

Make the sauce by mixing the vinegar, peanut butter, honey, mustard, soy
sauce, oils, broth, and orange juice. Use half the sauce to marinate the
scallops, turkey, and carrot for at least 1 hour.

Cook the vermicelli according to the package directions. Drain it well, and toss the pasta with the remaining half of the sauce, then heat it gently.

In a separate pan, heat the turkey and scallop mixture over low heat.

To serve, arrange the vermicelli in the center of a large platter, surround it with the turkey mixture, and sprinkle the sesame seeds and scallion on top.

Nutritional Analysis

Per Serving

Calories (kcal)	377.9	Cholesterol (mg)	51.0
Total Fat (g)	11.1	Dietary Fiber (g)	0.8
Saturated Fat (g)	2.3	% Calories from Fat	26.5
Monounsaturated Fat (g)	4.3	Vitamin C (mg)	6.0
Polyunsaturated Fat (g)	3.5	Vitamin A (i.u.)	3,482.0

SWEET-AND-SOUR CHICKEN
WITH VEGETABLES

This quickly prepared recipe offers a great way to use up leftovers, as any cooked meat, seafood, or poultry may be substituted for the cooked chicken. Although a very easy recipe, this dish has lots of flavor, color, and texture as well as a healthy dose of vitamins.

Makes 6 servings

1½ cups rice

1 tablespoon canola oil

3 medium carrots, sliced at an angle

1½ cups chopped yellow onion (bite-size pieces)

1½ cups chopped green bell pepper (bite-size pieces)

3 stalks celery, sliced at an angle

2 cups cooked chicken (bite-size pieces)

1 20-ounce can pineapple chunks in juice, drained

1 15-ounce can tomato sauce

½ cup water

¼ cup brown sugar

2 tablespoons fresh lemon juice

2 tablespoons low-sodium soy sauce

2 tablespoons rice wine vinegar

8 ounces low-fat tofu, cubed

Begin cooking the rice according to the package directions. While the rice is cooking, heat a large skillet to medium-high and pour the oil into the pan. Add the carrot and onion and sauté the vegetables for 5 minutes. Add the bell pepper and celery and cook 3 minutes longer, lowering the heat if necessary. Add the remaining ingredients, except the tofu, bring the contents to a boil, and boil gently for 3 minutes. Add the tofu and boil gently for 2 minutes longer.

Serve the chicken and vegetables over the hot rice.

Nutritional Analysis

Per Serving

Calories (kcal)	483.1	Cholesterol (mg)	40.0
Total Fat (g)	9.9	Dietary Fiber (g)	5.1
Saturated Fat (g)	2.1	% Calories from Fat	18.2
Monounsaturated Fat (g)	3.7	Vitamin C (mg)	41.0
Polyunsaturated Fat (g)	3.1	Vitamin A (i.u.)	9,941.0

Turkey in Tomatillo Sauce with Chili-Cilantro Waffles

Waffles that are not meant for breakfast, these are flecked with fresh cilantro and diced chilies to make a crisp and savory base for the delicious turkey in tomatillo sauce that gets spooned on top. Much more fun than rice or pasta.

Makes 6 servings

1 batch waffle batter (see below)

½ cup plus 3 tablespoons chopped fresh cilantro

⅓ cup plus 1½ tablespoons canned diced green chilies

1½ pounds cooked turkey breast meat

½ cup roasted pumpkin seeds (see below)

1 14-ounce can tomatillos, drained

2 cloves garlic, minced

3 large romaine lettuce leaves

6 tablespoons chopped yellow onion

1 cup low-fat chicken broth

½ teaspoon salt

¼ teaspoon cinnamon

⅛ teaspoon ground cloves

Prepare the waffles according to Veal with Shiitake Mushrooms over Lemon-Scallion Waffles (See Index), except omit the lemon zest and scallion and add, instead, the ½ cup cilantro and the ⅓ cup green chilies.

Cut the turkey into bite-size pieces and set it aside. If the pumpkin seeds are raw, toast them in a dry frying pan until they start to pop, about 5 minutes, and let them cool.

To make the sauce, combine the cooled seeds with the remaining ingredients in a blender or food processor and process until blended. Toss the sauce with the turkey and heat the mixture gently.

Serve the turkey-sauce mixture over the hot waffles.

Nutritional Analysis

Per Serving

Calories (kcal)	469.3	Cholesterol (mg)	156.0
Total Fat (g)	15.4	Dietary Fiber (g)	5.1
Saturated Fat (g)	3.6	% Calories from Fat	29.6
Monounsaturated Fat (g)	5.6	Vitamin C (mg)	23.0
Polyunsaturated Fat (g)	3.5	Vitamin A (i.u.)	429.0

TURKEY IN WHITE BEAN CHILI WITH CILANTRO CREAM

Everybody loves chili! The white beans and turkey not only set this dish apart from the traditional chili, but also give it a wonderfully delicious flavor and appeal. It boasts high fiber and low fat.

Makes 8 servings

1 pound white beans

1 tablespoon canola oil

2 cups chopped yellow onion

1 8-ounce can diced green chilies

6 cloves garlic, minced

1 teaspoon dried oregano

1½ teaspoons ground cumin

1 tablespoon chili powder

7 cups low-fat chicken broth

1 18-ounce can chopped tomatillos, drained*

1 cup plus 3 tablespoons chopped fresh cilantro, plus 8 fresh cilantro sprigs

1½ pounds skinless, boneless turkey breast, halved across

1 cup chopped scallion

2 tablespoons fresh lime juice

1 teaspoon salt

½ teaspoon white pepper

⅔ cup nonfat yogurt

3 tablespoons chopped fresh parsley

½ cup (3 ounces) grated cheddar cheese

Place the beans in a large bowl. Add enough cold water to cover the beans by at least 3 inches and let them soak for 8 to 12 hours.

Drain the beans. Heat the oil in a heavy pot over medium heat. Add the onion to the pot and sauté for 5 minutes. Add the chilies, garlic, oregano, cumin, and chili powder and sauté for another 5 minutes. Add the beans, broth, tomatillos, and the 1 cup chopped cilantro. Bring the bean mixture to a boil. Add the turkey and simmer the chili until the meat is just cooked through, about 20 minutes. Transfer the turkey to a plate. Allow the turkey to cool, then cover the plate with foil and refrigerate it. Continue simmering the chili until the beans are tender, about 2½ hours.

---

*Or use fresh tomatillos, chopped (about 3½ cups).

Cut the turkey into bite-size pieces. Add the turkey, scallion, and lime juice to the chili and stir to heat the contents through. Add the salt and white pepper (more or less, to taste).

Combine the yogurt, parsley, and remaining 3 tablespoons of chopped cilantro in a bowl to make the cilantro cream.

Ladle the chili into bowls. Top each with a spoonful of cilantro cream and a fresh cilantro sprig. Sprinkle each serving with grated cheese.

Nutritional Analysis

Per Serving

Calories (kcal)	444.4	Cholesterol (mg)	58.0
Total Fat (g)	11.5	Dietary Fiber (g)	11.8
Saturated Fat (g)	3.3	% Calories from Fat	21.3
Monounsaturated Fat (g)	3.8	Vitamin C (mg)	53.0
Polyunsaturated Fat (g)	2.0	Vitamin A (i.u.)	926.0

Turkey Scaloppine
with Lemon Cream Sauce

*The abundant lemon cream sauce tastes deceptively rich, with
a piquant flavor that adds great interest to usually bland turkey
and is a perfect complement to the broccoli. This colorful, delicious
recipe abounds with both vitamin C and beta-carotene.*

Makes 6 servings

2 cups low-fat chicken broth

1½ pounds turkey breast slices (6)

2 tablespoons butter

¼ cup flour

2 cups low-fat (1%) milk

6 tablespoons fresh lemon juice

1 teaspoon dried thyme

½ teaspoon salt

½ teaspoon pepper

6 cups steamed broccoli florets

1 cup finely chopped fresh parsley

1 teaspoon paprika

Bring the broth to a boil in a large skillet. Add the turkey and bring the broth to a second boil. Reduce the heat and simmer for 2 minutes, or until the meat is just cooked. Lift the turkey out of the broth, transfer it to a plate, and cover it to keep it warm.

In a clean skillet, melt the butter over high heat until it's foamy. Add the flour and whisk the mixture until blended. Turn the heat to the highest setting and immediately add the milk, whisking until the mixture comes to a boil. Reduce the heat to a simmer and add the lemon juice, thyme, salt, and pepper, whisking until smooth. Add the turkey, along with any accumulated juices, and the steamed broccoli to the pan and heat for 2 to 3 minutes, just until the turkey and broccoli are hot.

Dish up a slice of scaloppine on each plate, place some broccoli alongside it, and spoon extra sauce over both. Sprinkle each serving with the parsley and paprika.

Nutritional Analysis
Per Serving

Calories (kcal)	271.5	Cholesterol (mg)	60.0
Total Fat (g)	7.2	Dietary Fiber (g)	5.4
Saturated Fat (g)	3.6	% Calories from Fat	22.1
Monounsaturated Fat (g)	1.9	Vitamin C (mg)	127.0
Polyunsaturated Fat (g)	0.8	Vitamin A (i.u.)	3,266.0

MEAT

COOKING METHODS

Beef may be braised using the method for braising chicken suggested earlier in the chapter. However, the cooking time is longer: 2 hours. This method is particularly good for lean cuts of beef, such as top round or bottom round, which are the most economical. The meat can also be cut into thin strips and used in stir-fried dishes.

Sirloin tip may be broiled, cut into pieces for kabobs, or thinly sliced to create the base for a cold entree. Drizzle Ginger Sauce, Miso Dressing, or Mexican Green Chili Sauce from Chapter 8 over the beef and garnish it with radish florets and lime wedges.

If you're a meatloaf fan, try out Shiitake Mushroom Meatloaf, a light and delicious entree. Leftovers are great for sandwiches, and they don't have those surprise fat deposits you usually bite into in cold meatloaf.

In a hurry? Peppercorn Steaks with Noodles and Cabernet Sauce takes less than 30 minutes to prepare from the time you enter the kitchen.

As you can see, the recipes in this portion of the chapter offer many favorites with a flair, lowered fat content, and varied fusion-type dishes for every palate.

Irish Stew

This stew is very easy to make, forms a complete meal, and typifies any Irish grandmother's idea of good, plain cooking. Nothing complicated, just a hearty old-fashioned stew that is even better a day or two after it is made. We don't peel the potatoes for this stew—the skins add flavor, texture, vitamins, and fiber.

Makes 8 servings

3 pounds potatoes, chopped coarse

2 pounds yellow onions, chopped coarse

2 pounds carrots, chopped coarse

1 pound celery, chopped coarse

1½ pounds lean beef, cut into 1-inch cubes

¾ cup chopped fresh parsley

1½ teaspoons dried thyme

1 teaspoon salt

1 teaspoon pepper

2 cups low-fat beef broth

Preheat the oven to 250°F.

In a large, ovenproof casserole, layer one-third of the potatoes, one-third of the onions, one-third of the carrots, one-third of the celery, one-third of the beef, one-third of the parsley, and one-third of the thyme, salt, and pepper. Repeat the process, making two more layers. Pour the broth over the stew and cover the dish tightly. Bake the casserole for 2½ hours, then uncover the dish and bake for 1 hour longer. (The stew can also be simmered on top of the stove using the same procedure and cooking time.)

Before serving, stir the stew well.

Nutritional Analysis

Per Serving

Calories (kcal)	384.7	Cholesterol (mg)	52.0
Total Fat (g)	12.8	Dietary Fiber (g)	8.2
Saturated Fat (g)	5.0	% Calories from Fat	28.8
Monounsaturated Fat (g)	5.4	Vitamin C (mg)	53.0
Polyunsaturated Fat (g)	0.7	Vitamin A (i.u.)	28,785.0

Oven-Roasted Lamb
with Vegetable Sauce

This dish is fabulous and well worth the extra time.
It is a low-fat version of a Greek Island recipe.

Makes 10 servings

10 cups cooked white beans

2 pounds boneless leg of lamb, tied*

1½ teaspoons salt

¾ teaspoon pepper

3 carrots, chopped coarse

2 cloves garlic, sliced, plus 1 whole clove

1 large yellow onion, sliced

3 whole cloves

1 tablespoon olive oil

½ teaspoon dried thyme

1 bay leaf

2 tomatoes, peeled, seeded, and chopped

½ cup red wine

½ cup chopped fresh parsley

Preheat the oven to 400°F.

Rub the lamb with 1 teaspoon of the salt and ½ teaspoon of the pepper. Place it on a roasting pan and surround it with the carrot, sliced garlic, and onion slices stuck with the cloves. Drizzle the oil over the vegetables. Roast the pan at 400°F for 30 minutes, reduce the heat to 350°F and roast for 30 minutes more.

Remove the roasting pan from the oven and reduce the oven temperature to 225°F. Transfer the lamb to a casserole with a cover and add the remaining garlic clove, the thyme, the remaining ½ teaspoon of salt, the remaining ¼ teaspoon of pepper, the bay leaf, and the tomato. Add the vegetables from the roasting pan. Add the wine to the residue in the roasting pan and stir the mixture to incorporate any browned bits into the wine. Pour the wine mixture over the lamb. Cover the casserole tightly and cook it at 225°F for 5 hours.

---

*Lamb should weigh 2 pounds after fat is removed.

Transfer the lamb to a hot platter and remove any strings. Keep the lamb warm. Discard the bay leaf and the cloves from the onion. Skim off any fat, leaving the sauce and vegetables in the casserole. Over medium-high heat, boil the pan juices in the casserole for a few minutes, mashing the vegetables into the sauce. Sprinkle the sauce with the chopped parsley and serve it with the lamb.

Accompany the lamb with the cooked beans and some of the sauce spooned over them.

Nutritional Analysis

Per Serving

Calories (kcal)	465.0	Cholesterol (mg)	49.0
Total Fat (g)	14.8	Dietary Fiber (g)	10.8
Saturated Fat (g)	5.8	% Calories from Fat	28.5
Monounsaturated Fat (g)	6.1	Vitamin C (mg)	14.0
Polyunsaturated Fat (g)	1.4	Vitamin A (i.u.)	5,758.0

Peppercorn Steaks with Noodles and Cabernet Sauce

Double the recipe and serve this dish at a dinner party.

Makes 4 servings

2 teaspoons crushed black peppercorns

2 teaspoons green peppercorns in brine, drained

1 pound beef sirloin (4 fat-trimmed steaks)

1½ teaspoons olive oil

7 tablespoons brandy

⅓ cup finely chopped shallot

3 cloves garlic, minced

¾ cup dry red wine

2 teaspoons cornstarch

1 tablespoon water

12 ounces vermicelli

½ cup chopped fresh parsley

Peppercorn Steaks

Combine the black and green peppercorns and rub the mixture over both sides of the steaks. Heat the oil in a nonstick skillet over medium-high heat. Add the steaks and cook for 2½ minutes per side for medium-rare, or longer if desired. Remove the steaks from the pan and cover them lightly to keep them warm.

Cabernet Sauce

Add the brandy, shallot, and garlic to the pan and sauté the contents over medium-high heat for 2 minutes. Add the wine and boil the mixture until the liquid is slightly reduced (about 5 minutes). Combine the cornstarch and water; add the thickener to the simmering liquid in the pan and cook for about 3 minutes.

While making the sauce, cook the vermicelli according to the package directions, until just tender. Drain the pasta well.

Divide the pasta among four serving plates, top each portion with a steak, and spoon any accumulated juices over the meat. Top each serving with the parsley.

Nutritional Analysis

Per Serving

Calories (kcal)	663.0	Cholesterol (mg)	72.0
Total Fat (g)	18.3	Dietary Fiber (g)	0.4
Saturated Fat (g)	6.7	% Calories from Fat	29.0
Monounsaturated Fat (g)	8.2	Vitamin C (mg)	12.0
Polyunsaturated Fat (g)	0.8	Vitamin A (i.u.)	1,857.0

Shiitake Mushroom Meatloaf

This dish is versatile and scrumptious. When chilled and served the day after, it has the taste and texture of country-style pâté.

Makes 6 servings

¾ pound extra-lean ground beef

¼ cup oyster sauce

2 tablespoons low-sodium soy sauce

2 eggs, beaten

½ cup dry unseasoned bread crumbs

1 pound fresh shiitake mushrooms, chopped fine

½ cup finely chopped yellow onion

¼ teaspoon salt

¼ teaspoon pepper

Preheat the oven to 350°F.

Combine the beef with the oyster sauce, soy sauce, and eggs and mix until thoroughly combined and light in texture. Blend in the bread crumbs, again mixing until light. Add the mushrooms, onion, salt, and pepper and thoroughly combine all the ingredients. Place the mixture in a 9" × 5" × 3" loaf pan and bake for 1 hour.

Nutritional Analysis

Per Serving

Calories (kcal)	431.1	Cholesterol (mg)	104.0
Total Fat (g)	12.6	Dietary Fiber (g)	9.4
Saturated Fat (g)	4.7	% Calories from Fat	24.2
Monounsaturated Fat (g)	5.3	Vitamin C (mg)	4.0
Polyunsaturated Fat (g)	0.9	Vitamin A (i.u.)	90.0

Spicy Italian Sausages

*For a milder sausage, use only 1 teaspoon of the fennel seeds
and garlic powder and omit the crushed red pepper.*

Makes 8 servings

1 pound ground turkey breast

½ pound extra-lean ground
beef

¼ cup dry bread crumbs
(unseasoned)

½ cup low-fat (1%) milk

¼ cup dried onions

1½ teaspoons fennel seeds

1½ teaspoons garlic powder

1½ teaspoons dried oregano

1 teaspoon poultry seasoning

1 teaspoon crushed red pepper

1 large yellow onion, sliced

1 large green bell pepper, sliced

2 tablespoons water

1 16-ounce baguette, cut into 8
pieces

In a large bowl, combine the turkey, beef, bread crumbs, milk, dried onion,
and spices (through crushed red pepper); mix well. Shape the mixture into
eight sausages.

Separate the onion slices into rings. Coat a large nonstick frying pan with
cooking spray and place it over medium heat. When the pan is hot, add the
onion slices, bell pepper, and water. Cover the pan and cook the contents for
5 minutes, stirring occasionally, until the vegetables are fork-tender. Remove
the vegetables from the pan and cover them to keep them warm.

While the pan is still hot, add the sausages and cook, turning once, for
8 to 12 minutes, or until the meat is no longer pink in the center.

Split each piece of the baguette lengthwise and fill it with a sausage and slices
of the bell pepper and onion. Add mustard or other condiments as desired,
and serve.

Nutritional Analysis

Per Serving

Calories (kcal)	342.3	Cholesterol (mg)	53.0
Total Fat (g)	10.7	Dietary Fiber (g)	2.5
Saturated Fat (g)	3.4	% Calories from Fat	28.5
Monounsaturated Fat (g)	4.3	Vitamin C (mg)	10.0
Polyunsaturated Fat (g)	1.5	Vitamin A (i.u.)	120.0

Thai Beef and Mushroom Salad

Experiment with various mushroom varieties for different tastes.

Makes 8 servings

1 ounce dried shiitake or matsutake mushrooms

12 ounces flank steak

½ teaspoon freshly ground black pepper

½ pound bean sprouts, rinsed and drained

⅓ package (1¾-ounce package) bean threads (also called cellophane noodles)

½ pound zucchini, sliced diagonally

½ pound snow peas, halved diagonally

1 carrot, grated

1 small red onion, sliced thin

1 small green bell pepper, sliced thin

2 tablespoons soy sauce

½ teaspoon sugar

1 teaspoon hot chili oil

⅓ cup low-sodium beef broth

¼ cup rice wine vinegar

Cover the mushrooms with hot water and soak them for 30 minutes. Drain the mushrooms through a coffee filter, reserving the liquid. Squeeze the mushrooms dry, blot them with paper towels, and chop them.

Sprinkle the steak with the black pepper. Coat a nonstick frying pan with cooking spray, heat until it's very hot, and place the steak in the pan. Cook the steak for 4 minutes, then turn the steak over and cook it for 4 minutes more (or longer, if desired). Allow the meat to cool, then slice it thinly, on the diagonal, into bite-size pieces.

Combine the mushrooms, beef, bean sprouts, bean threads, zucchini, snow peas, carrot, onion, and bell pepper in a large bowl. Mix the remaining ingredients to make the dressing, whisking to combine them well.

Toss the dressing with the salad in a bowl.

Nutritional Analysis

Per Serving

Calories (kcal)	152.2	Cholesterol (mg)	22.0
Total Fat (g)	5.3	Dietary Fiber (g)	2.9
Saturated Fat (g)	2.0	% Calories from Fat	29.8
Monounsaturated Fat (g)	2.1	Vitamin C (mg)	28.0
Polyunsaturated Fat (g)	0.5	Vitamin A (i.u.)	2,436.0

Thyme-Crusted Pork Tenderloin

Pork has become leaner over the past decade. The tenderloin cut is low in fat but still tender and flavorful. This is another wonderful dinner-party dish.

Makes 8 servings

1¾ teaspoons pepper

1¾ teaspoons salt

1 tablespoon dried thyme

2 pounds pork tenderloin (may be in 2 pieces)

16 small red potatoes (about 2 pounds)

1 tablespoon olive oil

¼ cup fresh minced rosemary sprigs

½ cup chopped scallion

Preheat the oven to 350°F.

Combine 1½ teaspoons each of the pepper and salt and the 1 tablespoon thyme and sprinkle the mixture evenly over the pork, pressing the spices onto the surface. Place the meat on a rack in a roasting pan and bake for 1 hour to 1 hour and 20 minutes, depending on the thickness (until the internal temperature reaches 160°F). Remove the pan from the oven and raise the oven temperature to 400°F. Allow the juices to set for 5 to 10 minutes, then slice the meat on the bias.

Place the potatoes in a baking dish large enough to hold them in a single layer. Drizzle the oil over the potatoes and shake the pan to coat all sides of the potatoes. Sprinkle the potatoes with the remaining ¼ teaspoon each of salt and pepper and the rosemary, shaking the pan again to distribute the seasonings evenly. Bake the potatoes at 400°F for 45 minutes. (The potatoes may be baked with the pork for 1 hour, but they will not be as crisp as when baked at 400°F.)

When the potatoes have been baking for 30 minutes, put the pork slices back into the oven in a covered dish to reheat.

Sprinkle the potatoes with the scallion and serve them with the tenderloin.

Nutritional Analysis

Per Serving

Calories (kcal)	289.5	Cholesterol (mg)	74.0
Total Fat (g)	5.8	Dietary Fiber (g)	3.1
Saturated Fat (g)	1.6	% Calories from Fat	18.1
Monounsaturated Fat (g)	3.0	Vitamin C (mg)	38.0
Polyunsaturated Fat (g)	0.7	Vitamin A (i.u.)	53.0

Veal with Shiitake Mushrooms over Lemon-Scallion Waffles

Savory waffles studded with green onions and lemon zest cushion the delicate veal.

Makes 6 servings

1½ cups flour

2 tablespoons sugar

2 teaspoons baking powder

½ teaspoon baking soda

½ teaspoon salt

1 teaspoon white pepper

½ cup buttermilk

½ cup mineral water

2 tablespoons canola oil

2 egg yolks

4 egg whites

4 teaspoons lemon zest

1½ cups chopped scallion

1¼ pound veal cutlet, cut into ½-inch strips

1½ cups chopped yellow onion

1 teaspoon dried thyme

12 ounces chopped mushrooms

2 tablespoons brandy

2 cups low-fat chicken broth

½ cup (1 ounce) slivered sun-dried tomatoes

2 teaspoons cornstarch

1 tablespoon tap water

Lemon-Scallion Waffles

Coat a waffle iron with cooking spray and preheat it.

In a large bowl, combine the flour, sugar, baking powder, baking soda, salt, and ½ teaspoon of the white pepper. In a separate bowl, beat together the buttermilk, mineral water, 4 teaspoons of the oil, the egg yolks, lemon zest, and scallion. Mix the liquid with the dry ingredients. Beat the egg whites until they're stiff, then gently fold them into the batter.

Bake the waffles in the iron, using approximately ¾ cup batter for each, to desired crispness. The waffles may be made ahead and reheated briefly in a toaster or hot oven.

Veal

Coat a large skillet with cooking spray. Place the 2 remaining teaspoons of oil in the pan and set the heat to high. When the pan is hot, add the veal and cook for 5 minutes, tossing the meat constantly. Remove the veal and keep it warm.

Add the onion, thyme, and remaining pepper to the pan and cook for 3 minutes. Add the mushrooms and brandy and cook for 3 minutes more. Add the broth and sun-dried tomatoes and bring the mixture to a boil. Reduce the heat and simmer the contents for 5 minutes. Combine the cornstarch and tap water. Bring the mixture to a boil again and add the cornstarch mixture. Boil the sauce gently for 1 minute. Reduce the heat, return the veal to the pan, and simmer for 3 more minutes.

Serve the veal and mushroom sauce hot over the waffles.

Nutritional Analysis

Per Serving

Calories (kcal)	416.6	Cholesterol (mg)	151.0
Total Fat (g)	13.6	Dietary Fiber (g)	2.9
Saturated Fat (g)	8.7	% Calories from Fat	28.9
Monounsaturated Fat (g)	5.8	Vitamin C (mg)	19.0
Polyunsaturated Fat (g)	2.0	Vitamin A (i.u.)	260.0

Vegetarian Entrees

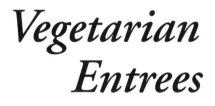

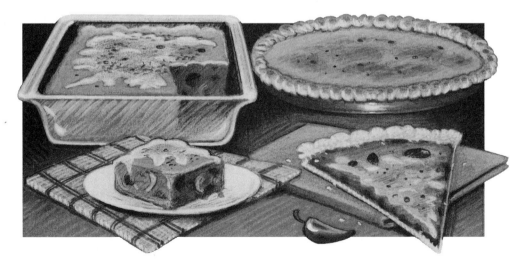

One easy way to reduce fat in your daily diet is to limit the number of servings of high-fat animal proteins. Health-conscious people have been doing this for years. Countless studies have linked vegetarian diets to a lower incidence of certain cancers. The Hindu population in India (vegetarians) have virtually no colon cancer. Seventh-Day Adventists in our country who are mainly vegetarians have a much lower incidence of all cancers, including colon, breast, lung, and esophageal.

Vegetarian dishes can provide all of your protein, vitamin, and mineral needs—and help assure you of good health. Whole grains, legumes, beans, rice, and vegetables are the mainstay of these dishes. Besides the benefit of low fat content, these entrees also contain a good amount of dietary fiber and vitamins. Low fat, high fiber, vitamin rich—it is no wonder meatless meals are so exceptional on a cancer risk-reduction eating plan.

There are so many delicious entrees made without high-fat animal protein. Because of their flavorful, rich taste and robust texture, they fulfill both your physical and psychological needs for food—there is something delicious to both chew and taste. And these meals are usually economical, a plus for the cost-conscious consumer.

When we published the first edition of this book, vegetarian meals were considered the domain of "health nuts." In the years since, many fabulous vegetarian cookbooks have been published because of public interest and demand.

Our goal in this chapter is to provide vegetarians with more exciting new dishes, and to introduce others to the versatility and satisfaction of a good meatless entree. This chapter was not written to try to convert you to vegetarianism. We merely want you to have good recipe choices if you are thinking of vegetarianism, or if you'd occasionally like to incorporate a meatless entree into your diet.

Plunging into a dietary regime that includes only plant foods (pure vegan) can be confusing if you don't know what you are doing. Before undertaking such a change, you may want to talk to your doctor or a registered dietitian (R.D.). Minerals, calcium, magnesium, iron, zinc, and iodine, as well as vitamin B_{12} supplement, brewer's yeast, and fortified cereal or soy milk are usually necessary for pure vegetarians.

On a lacto-ovo vegetarian diet (which includes plant foods, milk, other dairy products, and eggs), the risk of having a nutrient-deficient diet is minimal.

However, on this diet, it is easy to eat foods that are just as high in fat, saturated fat, and cholesterol as meat is. Hard cheese and eggs are the biggest offenders. One hard-cooked egg contains 250 milligrams of cholesterol and has 64 percent calories from fat. Hard cheeses such as Swiss, Monterey Jack, and cheddar contain about 73 percent calories from fat and 56 milligrams of cholesterol per 2-ounce serving. The maximum daily intake for cholesterol recommended by the American Heart Association is 300 milligrams.

Many Americans already eat vegetarian meals without even realizing it. These include manicotti (ricotta cheese with grain), pizza (part-skim cheese with a grain crust), Spanish rice and beans, macaroni and cheese, and bean burritos (beans and a corn or wheat tortilla). We will show you how to make low-fat versions of these recipes, since the standard versions of many of these favorite foods contain well over 30 percent calories from fat.

Some of the ingredients in vegetarian entrees are incomplete proteins (that is, they don't contain all essential amino acids) by themselves. But when eaten in certain combinations, they become complete protein sources, contributing all nine essential amino acids. See the Appendix for a simple chart on combining proteins to make "complete" proteins.

A very popular combination that offers complete protein is rice and beans. Combining these two food staples has kept many civilizations healthy and thriving throughout the centuries. Brazilian Black Beans and Rice is delicious. Serve this dish with a tangy green salad. Or try Mexican Rice-Crust Pizza. This is a perfect children's party meal.

Quiche is still a favorite for brunch or a light supper. We have a wonderful Spinach and Feta Herb Quiche in which we mix two low-fat cheeses together. This recipe demonstrates how cheese can fit into a cancer risk-reduction diet.

Chili-Cheese Pie is another exceptional brunch dish. It contains good amounts of protein and 16.1 grams of fiber, which is almost one-half of your daily fiber requirement.

There are many more tasty and varied recipes in this chapter. We have highlighted some of them to show how healthful ingredients make good-tasting meatless entrees. We are sure you will discover your own favorites.

Spicy Thai Tofu is a great introduction to the myriad possibilities of using soy products as a cancer prevention food. As we mentioned in the Introduction, the evidence linking soy products to reduced cancer risk is mounting.

Bean Cakes are quick, easy, and low in calories as well as containing more than 17 grams of fiber per serving.

Bulgur and Pepper Bake is a perfect company meal when you want something a little unusual. Serve this dish with Middle Eastern bread (lavrosh) and our Greek Yogurt-Dill Sauce as a dip (see Chapter 8).

We can't emphasize enough the importance of dietary fiber. The recipes in this chapter are exemplary in their fiber content. They demonstrate how simple it can be to attain the 35 grams recommended for daily consumption.

Bean Cakes

This is the ultimate recipe for those occasions when you have nothing fresh in the refrigerator. The ingredients are likely to be on hand, and the cakes are lightly crispy and delicious. Serve them alone or, if you have the condiments and want to take a little more time, also offer avocado, salsa, light sour cream, chopped green onions, part-skim mozzarella, baked tortilla chips, or any other garnishes you might have around.

Makes 8 servings

3 cups canned kidney beans, drained

¼ teaspoon cayenne

2 cloves garlic, minced

½ teaspoon salt

1 tablespoon butter

1 tablespoon olive oil

Chop the beans coarsely, then add the cayenne, garlic, and salt. Mix until the ingredients are well combined. With your hands, form the mixture into eight flat cakes. Place the butter and oil in a skillet and sauté the cakes over medium heat for 5 minutes on each side, or until they're golden brown.

Nutritional Analysis

Per Serving

Calories (kcal)	258.4	Cholesterol (mg)	4.0
Total Fat (g)	3.7	Dietary Fiber (g)	17.2
Saturated Fat (g)	1.2	% Calories from Fat	12.5
Monounsaturated Fat (g)	1.7	Vitamin C (mg)	3.0
Polyunsaturated Fat (g)	0.5	Vitamin A (i.u.)	82.0

Brazilian Black Beans and Rice

Vegan recipe *(no meat or dairy), without the use of yogurt as a condiment.*

Makes 6 servings

1 pound black beans
1 cup brown rice
1 tablespoon vegetable oil
1 cup chopped yellow onion
3 cloves garlic, minced
½ teaspoon salt
¼ teaspoon pepper
1 tablespoon olive oil
1 tablespoon red wine vinegar

Condiments

1 cup finely chopped yellow onion
1½ cups salsa
1 avocado, chopped
6 tablespoons chopped fresh cilantro
¾ cup nonfat yogurt

Soak the beans for 8 to 12 hours in enough water to cover them. Drain the beans and place them in a pot, again with just enough water to cover them. Cook the beans over low heat for 2 hours, or until they're tender. Then drain them.

Start cooking the rice according to the package directions.

Heat the vegetable oil in a skillet, add the 1 cup chopped onion and the garlic, and sauté the vegetables until they're soft, about 5 minutes. Add ½ cup of the cooked beans and mash them into the onion mixture until they are almost smooth. Add the remaining beans and simmer the mixture for about 30 minutes or until it's thickened. Add the salt, pepper, olive oil, and vinegar, stirring to combine.

Serve the beans over the hot rice, with the condiments in bowls for each individual to add as desired.

Nutritional Analysis

Per Serving

Calories (kcal)	617.5	Cholesterol (mg)	1.0
Total Fat (g)	13.8	Dietary Fiber (g)	16.4
Saturated Fat (g)	2.0	% Calories from Fat	19.5
Monounsaturated Fat (g)	6.8	Vitamin C (mg)	24.0
Polyunsaturated Fat (g)	2.9	Vitamin A (i.u.)	852.0

BROCCOLI QUICHE

*This is delicious—for breakfast, lunch, or dinner. We also cut it into
small squares and serve it as an appetizer. Make one or two
during the holidays; you never know who will drop in.*

Makes 8 servings

2 pounds broccoli florets

½ cup flour

4 eggs, beaten

4 ounces grated mozzarella
cheese, part skim

4 cups low-fat (2%) cottage
cheese

½ cup finely chopped fresh
parsley

½ red onion, minced

2 cloves garlic, minced

2 tablespoons fresh lemon juice

1 teaspoon dried oregano

1 teaspoon chopped fresh basil

1 teaspoon salt

½ teaspoon pepper

⅔ cup dry seasoned bread
crumbs

Preheat the oven to 350°F. Coat a 9" × 13" pan with cooking spray.

Steam the broccoli florets until they're just tender, then drain them and chop
them coarsely. In a large bowl, whisk the flour with the eggs. Add the broccoli
and all the remaining ingredients, except the bread crumbs. Mix the ingredients gently but thoroughly.

Place the broccoli mixture in the pan, then sprinkle the bread crumbs on top.
Bake the quiche for 35 to 40 minutes.

Let the quiche cool for 5 minutes, then cut it into bars to serve.

Nutritional Analysis

Per Serving

Calories (kcal)	278.8	Cholesterol (mg)	109.0
Total Fat (g)	7.5	Dietary Fiber (g)	4.0
Saturated Fat (g)	3.7	% Calories from Fat	23.9
Monounsaturated Fat (g)	2.3	Vitamin C (mg)	85.0
Polyunsaturated Fat (g)	0.7	Vitamin A (i.u.)	2,151.0

BULGUR AND PEPPER BAKE

This is a special treat if you have never tried bulgur. It is a wonderful food—high in fiber, tasty, and satisfying.

Makes 8 servings

1½ cups bulgur cracked wheat

1 tablespoon canola oil

1 tablespoon vegetable broth

1½ cups chopped yellow onion

4 cups chopped green bell pepper

1½ cups sliced mushrooms

1½ tablespoons sherry (or broth)

1 teaspoon dried oregano

½ teaspoon salt

¼ teaspoon black pepper

2 ounces crumbled feta cheese

1½ cups low-fat (2%) cottage cheese

4 eggs, beaten

½ teaspoon paprika

Soak the bulgur in 1½ cups water for 30 minutes, then drain it well.

Preheat the oven to 350°F. Coat a 9" × 13" pan with cooking spray.

In a large skillet, combine the oil and broth, then add the onion and sauté the mixture over medium heat until the onion is translucent. Add the bell pepper and mushrooms and cook until the pepper is almost tender. Remove the pan from the heat. Add the sherry, oregano, salt, and black pepper and mix well.

Combine the feta cheese with the cottage cheese. Spread the drained bulgur over the bottom of the pan and cover the bulgur with the vegetables, then with the mixed cheeses. Pour the eggs over the top and sprinkle it with the paprika. Bake for 40 minutes.

Let the pan set for 10 minutes before cutting and serving.

Nutritional Analysis

Per Serving

Calories (kcal)	225.1	Cholesterol (mg)	101.0
Total Fat (g)	6.8	Dietary Fiber (g)	7.6
Saturated Fat (g)	2.5	% Calories from Fat	26.4
Monounsaturated Fat (g)	2.4	Vitamin C (mg)	39.0
Polyunsaturated Fat (g)	1.1	Vitamin A (i.u.)	581.0

California Baked Beans

This is our version of pork and beans, without the high fat content in the usual canned variety.

Makes 6 servings

1 tablespoon olive oil

2 cups chopped yellow onion

1 cup chopped green bell pepper

2 teaspoons chili powder

1 teaspoon Dijon mustard

½ teaspoon salt

½ teaspoon black pepper

2 tablespoons brown sugar

6 ounces grated mozzarella cheese, part skim

2 cups chopped tomato

¼ cup dry white wine (or broth)

3 15-ounce cans pinto beans, drained

Preheat the oven to 350°F. Coat a large casserole with cooking spray.

Heat the oil in a large skillet. Add the onion and bell pepper and sauté the vegetables for 5 minutes. Add the chili powder, mustard, salt, black pepper, and brown sugar and stir the mixture to combine the ingredients well. Remove the pan from the heat and add the cheese, tomato, and wine; stir in the beans.

Transfer the mixture to the casserole. Cover the dish and bake the beans for 45 minutes.

Serve hot.

Nutritional Analysis

Per Serving

Calories (kcal)	261.1	Cholesterol (mg)	15.0
Total Fat (g)	8.0	Dietary Fiber (g)	6.6
Saturated Fat (g)	3.5	% Calories from Fat	27.6
Monounsaturated Fat (g)	3.2	Vitamin C (mg)	32.0
Polyunsaturated Fat (g)	0.6	Vitamin A (i.u.)	1,055.0

CHEESE ENCHILADAS
WITH GREEN SAUCE

*This is a delicious alternative to standard high-fat enchiladas, with a creamy
filling and a flavorful sauce. It has 97 percent of the RDA of vitamin C
and 35 percent of the RDA of vitamin A (beta-carotene).*

Makes 8 servings

3 cups low-fat (1%) cottage
  cheese

½ cup chopped fresh parsley

1½ teaspoons dried thyme

1½ teaspoons dried oregano

½ teaspoon salt

1 12-ounce can diced green
  chilies

1½ cups vegetable broth (or
  chicken broth)

10 large romaine lettuce leaves,
  torn into pieces

1 tablespoon canola oil

8 flour tortillas

4 ounces grated mozzarella
  cheese, part skim

Preheat the oven to 400°F.

Mix the cottage cheese, parsley, thyme, oregano, and salt to make the filling.

To make the sauce, process the chilies, broth, and lettuce in a food processor
or blender until the mixture is smooth. Heat the oil in a skillet, add the sauce,
and simmer for 5 minutes.

Soften the tortillas by heating them on a griddle or in a frying pan. Fill the
tortillas with the cottage cheese mixture and roll them up. Pour half of the
sauce into a 9" × 13" pan and add the filled tortillas, seam-side down. Cover
the tortillas with the remaining sauce and sprinkle them with the grated
cheese. Bake the enchiladas for 20 minutes.

Serve hot.

Nutritional Analysis

Per Serving

Calories (kcal)	278.2	Cholesterol (mg)	12.0
Total Fat (g)	8.5	Dietary Fiber (g)	2.3
Saturated Fat (g)	2.8	% Calories from Fat	27.6
Monounsaturated Fat (g)	3.2	Vitamin C (mg)	58.0
Polyunsaturated Fat (g)	1.9	Vitamin A (i.u.)	1,709.0

CHILI-CHEESE PIE

This is similar to a tamale pie, but with a tasty cornmeal crust holding the filling. This is another great dish for a children's party. Serve it with a platter of raw vegetables.

Makes 8 servings

2½ cups water

1 teaspoon salt

1 teaspoon chili powder

1⅓ cups cornmeal

1 tablespoon canola oil

½ cup chopped yellow onion

½ cup chopped green bell pepper

1 4-ounce can diced green chilies

1 teaspoon dried oregano

½ teaspoon ground cumin

¼ teaspoon black pepper

1 15-ounce can kidney beans, drained

½ cup frozen corn, defrosted and drained

4 ounces grated mozzarella cheese, part skim

2 ounces grated cheddar cheese

1 egg, beaten

¼ cup low-fat (1%) milk

2 medium tomatoes, sliced thin

Cornmeal Piecrust

Combine the water, ½ teaspoon of the salt, ½ teaspoon of the chili powder, and the cornmeal in a saucepan and cook the mixture over medium heat until it becomes stiff (about 10 minutes), stirring frequently. Coat a 9" × 13" dish with cooking spray, and line the sides and bottom with the cornmeal mixture.

Chili-Cheese Filling

Heat the oil in a large skillet. Add the onion, bell pepper, and chilies and sauté the vegetables for 5 minutes over medium heat. Add the oregano, cumin, the remaining ½ teaspoon chili powder, the remaining ½ teaspoon salt, and the black pepper. Remove the pan from the heat and add the drained beans and corn.

Preheat the oven to 350°F.

Combine the two cheeses. In a separate bowl, mix the egg and milk. Add the liquid to the bean mixture along with one-third of the cheese mixture. Spread another third of the cheese mixture over the bottom of the crust. Spoon in the bean filling and press it down gently. Arrange the sliced tomato over the filling and sprinkle the remaining third of the cheese mixture over the top. Bake the pie for 35 minutes.

Allow the pie to cool for 5 to 10 minutes before cutting and serving.

Nutritional Analysis

Per Serving

Calories (kcal)	385.6	Cholesterol (mg)	38.0
Total Fat (g)	8.3	Dietary Fiber (g)	16.1
Saturated Fat (g)	2.7	% Calories from Fat	19.0
Monounsaturated Fat (g)	3.1	Vitamin C (mg)	32.0
Polyunsaturated Fat (g)	0.09	Vitamin A (i.u.)	777.0

Eggplant Parmesan

The eggplant slices are baked, rather than fried in oil—which eliminates the usual high amount of fat.

Makes 8 servings

3 medium eggplants, peeled

½ teaspoon salt, plus extra salt for the eggplant

2 teaspoons olive oil

1½ cups finely chopped yellow onion

2 cloves garlic, minced

2 cups low-fat (2%) cottage cheese

3 ounces grated mozzarella cheese, part skim

½ cup dry unseasoned bread crumbs

1 teaspoon dried oregano

1 teaspoon chopped fresh basil

1 teaspoon dried thyme

¼ teaspoon pepper

3 tomatoes, sliced thin

2 cups marinara sauce (low-fat)

1 ounce grated Parmesan cheese

Preheat oven to 350°F. Coat a baking tray and a 9" × 13" pan with cooking spray.

Slice the eggplants and salt the slices lightly. (Salting the eggplant helps to draw out excess moisture.) Place the eggplant slices on the baking tray and bake them for 15 minutes, or until they're tender.

Heat the oil in a skillet over medium heat. Add the onion and garlic and sauté the vegetables until they're soft. Remove the pan from the heat and add the cottage cheese, mozzarella, bread crumbs, oregano, basil, thyme, the ½ teaspoon of salt, and the pepper.

Layer half of the baked eggplant slices in the pan. Spread the cheese mixture over the eggplant. Top the cheese with the remaining eggplant slices. Place the tomato slices on top of the eggplant. Pour the marinara sauce over the tomato layer and sprinkle the Parmesan over the sauce. Cover the pan and bake for 25 minutes; uncover and bake for 10 minutes more.

Let the dish set a few minutes before serving.

Nutritional Analysis

Per Serving

Calories (kcal)	240.1	Cholesterol (mg)	13.0
Total Fat (g)	8.1	Dietary Fiber (g)	5.0
Saturated Fat (g)	3.2	% Calories from Fat	28.7
Monounsaturated Fat (g)	3.3	Vitamin C (mg)	20.0
Polyunsaturated Fat (g)	1.0	Vitamin A (i.u.)	1,204.0

Lentil Fritters with Spiced Yogurt Dip

Vegan recipe (no meat or dairy), without the yogurt dip.

*This East Indian dish with its unique blend of spices makes
a wonderful appetizer, light entree, or side dish.*

Makes 6 servings (about 30 fritters)

1 cup dried lentils

1 cup nonfat yogurt

4 teaspoons olive oil, plus
  additional as needed for
  frying

½ teaspoon ground cumin

½ teaspoon dried oregano

¼ teaspoon chili powder

¾ teaspoon salt

4½ tablespoons flour

2 tablespoons canned, diced
  green chilies

Cook the lentils according to the package directions; drain them well and let
them cool to room temperature.

While the lentils are cooling prepare the dip. In a small bowl, combine the
yogurt, 1 teaspoon of the oil, the cumin, oregano, chili powder, and ¼ teaspoon of the salt.

To make the fritters, in a food processor or blender, process the cooled lentils,
flour, chilies, and the remaining ½ teaspoon of salt until the mixture is
smooth. Brush a griddle or heavy frying pan with 1 tablespoon of the remaining oil and heat the pan to medium-high. Place tablespoon-size portions of
the lentil mixture in the hot pan and fry them for 1 minute. Turn them over,
press the mounds gently to flatten them, and fry them for 2 minutes more.
The fritters should be round and flat. Brush the pan with more oil, as needed,
and continue frying the lentil mixture in batches. Cover the cooked fritters to
keep them warm while the remaining fritters are being fried.

Serve the warm fritters with the spiced yogurt dip.

Nutritional Analysis

Per Serving

Calories (kcal)	180.2	Cholesterol (mg)	1.0
Total Fat (g)	3.6	Dietary Fiber (g)	10.0
Saturated Fat (g)	0.5	% Calories from Fat	17.4
Monounsaturated Fat (g)	2.3	Vitamin C (mg)	6.0
Polyunsaturated Fat (g)	0.4	Vitamin A (i.u.)	83.0

Mexican Rice-Crust Pizza

This wonderful "pizza" is packed with flavor. The crust is made with brown rice, which adds fiber. It contains only a bit of the usual fat that is commonly present in pizza.

Makes 8 servings

3 cups cooked brown rice

3 ounces grated mozzarella cheese, part skim

2 eggs, beaten

1 cup chopped, cooked kidney beans, drained

1 14-ounce can tomatillos, drained

⅓ cup finely chopped yellow onion

2 cloves garlic, minced

1 4-ounce can diced green chilies

⅓ cup chopped fresh cilantro

1 teaspoon sugar

½ teaspoon salt

3 ounces grated Monterey Jack cheese

½ cup sliced green bell pepper

½ cup sliced mushrooms

½ cup sliced tomato

¼ cup sliced scallion

Preheat the oven to 375°F.

Brown Rice Pizza Crust

Coat a 9" × 13" baking pan with cooking spray. Combine the rice, mozzarella, and eggs and spread the mixture in the pan. Spread the chopped beans over the rice mixture.

Tomatillo Sauce

Combine the tomatillos, onion, garlic, chilies, cilantro, sugar, and salt in a food processor or blender and process the mixture until smooth. Spread the sauce over the beans. Sprinkle the pizza with the grated cheese and the remaining toppings.

Bake the pizza for 40 minutes. Let the pizza cool for a few minutes, then cut it into bars and serve.

Nutritional Analysis

Per Serving

Calories (kcal)	227.0	Cholesterol (mg)	61.0
Total Fat (g)	7.5	Dietary Fiber (g)	3.9
Saturated Fat (g)	3.7	% Calories from Fat	29.3
Monounsaturated Fat (g)	2.1	Vitamin C (mg)	32.0
Polyunsaturated Fat (g)	0.6	Vitamin A (i.u.)	510.0

SAUTÉED VEGETABLES
WITH PASTA AND GREENS

Vegan recipe (no meat or dairy), if vegetable broth is used
instead of chicken broth, and the cheese is omitted as a topping.

Makes 6 servings

3 cups frozen black-eyed peas
(1 pound)

1½ tablespoons olive oil

2 cups peeled and chopped
jicama

1⅓ cups chopped green, red, or
yellow bell pepper

½ cup chopped carrot

½ cup chopped yellow onion

4 cloves garlic, minced

1 8-ounce can tomato sauce

¾ cup low-fat chicken broth

¼ cup chopped fresh oregano

¼ cup chopped fresh cilantro

10 ounces bow-tie pasta

6 ounces baby lettuce or mixed
greens

3 tablespoons freshly grated
Parmesan cheese

Cook the black-eyed peas in a medium-size pot of boiling water until they're just tender, about 30 minutes. Drain the peas.

Heat the oil in a heavy, large skillet over medium-high heat. Add the jicama, bell pepper, carrot, onion, and garlic, and sauté the vegetables for 5 minutes. Add the tomato sauce, broth, oregano, cilantro, and drained black-eyed peas and bring the mixture to a boil. Reduce the heat and simmer the sauce for 10 minutes, stirring occasionally.

Meanwhile, cook the pasta in a large pot of boiling salted water until it's just tender but still firm to the bite, stirring occasionally. Drain the pasta well.

Divide the lettuce among the serving plates. Top each serving with one-sixth of the pasta and the vegetable sauce. Sprinkle each portion with ½ tablespoon of the cheese and serve.

Nutritional Analysis

Per Serving

Calories (kcal)	393.6	Cholesterol (mg)	2.0
Total Fat (g)	6.1	Dietary Fiber (g)	10.2
Saturated Fat (g)	1.2	% Calories from Fat	13.6
Monounsaturated Fat (g)	2.9	Vitamin C (mg)	37.0
Polyunsaturated Fat (g)	1.0	Vitamin A (i.u.)	3,219.0

SPICY THAI TOFU

Vegan recipe *(no meat or dairy)*.

This dish has a wonderful flavor—a vegetarian dish that will appeal to everyone!

Makes 4 servings

¼ cup fresh lemon juice

¼ cup fresh lime juice

⅓ cup chopped fresh Italian parsley

⅓ cup chopped fresh cilantro

2 tablespoons chopped fresh mint

½ cup low-sodium soy sauce

2 tablespoons peanut butter

1 tablespoon finely minced fresh ginger

1 tablespoon sesame oil (Asian variety)

½ teaspoon red pepper flakes

3 cloves garlic, minced

21 ounces firm, reduced-fat tofu

12 ounces soba noodles or other thin pasta

To make the marinade, combine all the ingredients except the tofu and pasta in a food processor or blender and process them well. Cut the tofu into eight pieces. Place the pieces in the marinade, cover the container, and marinate the tofu for 1 hour. Turn the pieces over and marinate them at least 1 hour longer.

Cook the pasta according to the package directions. Drain it, transfer it to a large bowl, and cover it to keep it warm until the tofu is cooked.

Coat a nonstick skillet or griddle with cooking spray and heat it to medium-high. Remove the tofu pieces from the marinade, reserving the liquid. Place the tofu in the skillet and cook the pieces for 2 minutes on each side, or until they're golden brown. Remove the tofu from the skillet and cover the pieces to keep them warm. Pour the marinade into the skillet and bring it to a boil. Pour the warm marinade over the pasta and toss the mixture to combine well.

Dish up the pasta, topping each serving with two slices of cooked tofu.

Nutritional Analysis

Per Serving

Calories (kcal)	540.5	Cholesterol (mg)	0.0
Total Fat (g)	16.8	Dietary Fiber (g)	7.6
Saturated Fat (g)	2.6	% Calories from Fat	25.8
Monounsaturated Fat (g)	5.3	Vitamin C (mg)	20.0
Polyunsaturated Fat (g)	7.7	Vitamin A (i.u.)	459.0

SPINACH AND FETA HERB QUICHE

This recipe may be halved and baked in one pie plate. However, this dish is so versatile—serve it as an entree, a lunch dish, an appetizer when cut in small pieces, or a great picnic item—that you'll want to keep one in the freezer. It is a low-calorie entree as well.

Makes 12 servings (2 quiches)

1 tablespoon olive oil

1½ cups chopped yellow onion

4 teaspoons flour

1 teaspoon salt

1 teaspoon dried oregano

1 teaspoon dried thyme

½ teaspoon garlic powder

½ teaspoon pepper

3 cups low-fat (1%) milk

4 cups cooked rice (1½ cups raw)

3 ounces crumbled feta cheese

2 eggs plus 4 egg whites, beaten

1 20-ounce package frozen spinach, defrosted and squeezed dry

¼ cup grated Romano or Asiago cheese

Preheat the oven to 400°F. Coat two pie plates with cooking spray.

Heat a large skillet to medium hot and pour the oil into the pan. When the oil is hot, add the onion and sauté it for 3 minutes. Add the flour, salt, oregano, thyme, garlic powder, and pepper and stir the mixture to blend the ingredients. Add the milk and bring the contents to a boil, whisking constantly. Reduce the heat and simmer the mixture for 2 minutes, until it's a bit thickened, again whisking constantly.

Remove the pan from the heat. Add the cooked rice, feta, eggs and whites, and spinach, stirring to combine well. Divide the mixture between the two pie plates. Sprinkle each pie with the grated cheese and bake them for 30 minutes.

Serve slices of quiche hot or chilled.

Nutritional Analysis

Per Serving

Calories (kcal)	184.4	Cholesterol (mg)	42.0
Total Fat (g)	5.0	Dietary Fiber (g)	2.1
Saturated Fat (g)	2.3	% Calories from Fat	24.4
Monounsaturated Fat (g)	1.9	Vitamin C (mg)	13.0
Polyunsaturated Fat (g)	0.4	Vitamin A (i.u.)	3,894.0

SPINACH-CHEESE PANCAKES

These are packed with vitamins—233 percent of the RDA of vitamin A (beta-carotene) and 71 percent of the RDA of vitamin C! This dish also supplies a good amount of calcium.

Makes 4 servings

2 eggs, beaten

1½ teaspoons olive oil

1¾ cups low-fat (1%) milk

1 20-ounce package frozen spinach, defrosted and squeezed dry

4 ounces grated mozzarella cheese, part skim

½ cup sliced scallion plus 2 tablespoons minced scallion

¾ teaspoon salt

1 teaspoon dried oregano

¼ teaspoon sugar

½ teaspoon pepper

1 cup flour

1 cup nonfat yogurt

Spinach-Cheese Pancakes

Combine the eggs, oil, and milk. Add the spinach and combine it thoroughly with the milk mixture. Add the cheese, the ½ cup sliced scallion, ½ teaspoon of the salt, ½ teaspoon of the oregano, the sugar, and ¼ teaspoon of the pepper and mix. Add the flour and combine until the ingredients are well blended.

Coat a skillet or griddle with cooking spray. Using approximately 2 tablespoons batter for each pancake, fry the cakes until they're golden and crispy on both sides.

Oregano Sauce

Combine the yogurt with the remaining ½ teaspoon oregano, ¼ teaspoon salt, ¼ teaspoon pepper, and the minced scallion.

Serve the sauce with the hot pancakes.

Nutritional Analysis

Per Serving

Calories (kcal)	358.0	Cholesterol (mg)	112.0
Total Fat (g)	10.7	Dietary Fiber (g)	5.7
Saturated Fat (g)	4.9	% Calories from Fat	26.5
Monounsaturated Fat (g)	3.8	Vitamin C (mg)	43.0
Polyunsaturated Fat (g)	1.0	Vitamin A (i.u.)	11,619.0

WHITE BEAN–TOMATILLO CHILI WITH CILANTRO-CREAM SALSA

Vegan recipe (no meat or dairy), if vegetable broth is used instead of chicken broth, and the cilantro-cream salsa is omitted.

This recipe uses 1 tablespoon oil to sauté the onion, chilies, garlic, and spices. Often with a multi-ingredient dish, sautéing can be omitted, but with this chili we want to bring out the intensity of the seasonings, so we use 1 tablespoon oil for a dish that serves six people. Each serving has half the recommended grams of daily dietary fiber.

Makes 6 servings

1 pound white beans

1 tablespoon canola oil

2 cups chopped yellow onion

1 8-ounce can diced green chilies

6 cloves garlic, minced

1½ tablespoons dried oregano

1 tablespoon ground cumin

1 tablespoon chili powder

7 cups low-fat chicken broth

1 24-ounce can tomatillos, drained and chopped

1¼ cups chopped fresh cilantro plus 6 cilantro sprigs

1 cup chopped scallion

1 tablespoon fresh lime juice

⅔ cup nonfat yogurt

⅓ cup light sour cream

⅓ cup salsa

⅓ cup chopped fresh parsley

White Bean Chili

Place the beans in a large bowl and add enough water to cover them by several inches. Allow the beans to set for 8 to 12 hours. Drain the beans.

Heat the oil in a large skillet. Add the onion and sauté over medium heat for 5 minutes. Add the chilies, garlic, oregano, cumin, and chili powder and sauté the mixture for 5 minutes longer. Add the beans, broth, tomatillos, and 1 cup of the chopped cilantro. Bring the mixture to a boil, reduce the heat, and let the mixture simmer for 3 hours, stirring occasionally. Add the scallion and lime juice and stir to heat through.

Cilantro-Cream Salsa

Combine the yogurt, sour cream, salsa, parsley, and the remaining ¼ cup chopped cilantro.

Pour a spoonful of salsa on top of each serving of chili and garnish with a cilantro sprig.

Nutritional Analysis

Per Serving

Calories (kcal)	411.0	Cholesterol (mg)	1.0
Total Fat (g)	5.8	Dietary Fiber (g)	16.4
Saturated Fat (g)	0.4	% Calories from Fat	11.0
Monounsaturated Fat (g)	1.4	Vitamin C (mg)	79.0
Polyunsaturated Fat (g)	1.1	Vitamin A (i.u.)	1,380.0

Vegetables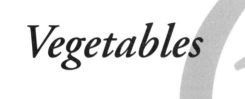

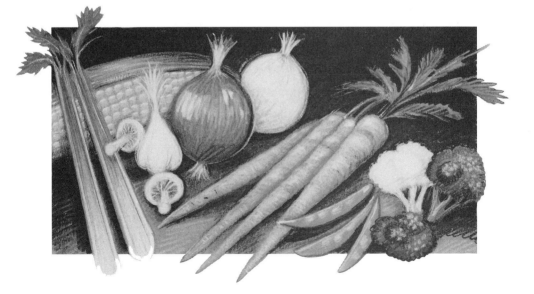

Eat More Vegetables!

As a part of a cancer risk-reduction eating plan, vegetables provide an eye-catching array of nature's bounty: colorful leafy spinach, sweet baby carrots, bright broccoli florets, luscious beefsteak tomatoes. These vegetables gratify our senses and keep us healthy. Plain or fancy, steamed, sautéed, stir-fried, or baked, they rank among the best foods, and we simply must eat more.

Whenever possible, we use fresh, homegrown (farmer's market) fruits and vegetables. Their taste and appealing texture make any dish a masterpiece. Living in Sonoma County, California, Terri Pischoff has the luxury of year-round locally grown organic produce. However, across the country many people spend weekend mornings strolling through local farmer's markets. If you have not had this experience yet, you will be pleasantly surprised. It is a relaxing way to spend a morning.

Fruits and vegetables play an extremely important role in protecting the body from certain cancers. The most significant of the vegetables are those high in beta-carotene and vitamin C. Vegetables high in beta-carotene come in two colors: yellow-orange and dark green. Vegetables with the darkest colors tend to contain the most beta-carotene. Carrots, sweet potatoes, pumpkin, and winter squash stand out in the yellow-orange group; Swiss chard, spinach, broccoli, kale, and turnip greens top the list of the dark green group.

People who eat large amounts of green and yellow vegetables have a lower incidence of certain cancers. Two decades ago, the cancer rates in Japan were significantly lower than those of the United States or Northern Europe. Since the "westernization" of their diets (higher fat and fewer fruits and vegetables), their cancer rates are now comparable to those of the United States.

Broccoli, cabbage, brussels sprouts, green peppers, potatoes, and most dark green leafy vegetables all contain good amounts of vitamin C. Cabbage, kale, brussels sprouts, turnips, mustard and turnip greens, and cauliflower, are also a good source of vitamins C and A (beta-carotene).

This chapter shows you many ways to prepare these wonderfully healthful vegetables. We use fresh vegetables in most of the recipes—they are certainly tastier and more attractive than packaged ones. But sometimes the frozen variety is all that is available or convenient. Frozen vegetables do have this advantage: they can be stored for weeks and used when needed, and methods of quick freezing usually ensure maximum vitamin content.

For the sake of keeping fat intake per meal to no more than 30 percent, use the simple rule of *plain entree/fancy vegetable.* Applying this rule gives you leeway with salad dressings and side dishes. If you are planning a low-fat entree, you have room to enjoy some of our creamy vegetable dishes, or those made with a little more oil or butter. Even these vegetable dishes are low in fat (if you maintain portion size!).

Begin with some of the simplest vegetable dishes: Garlic-Sautéed Spinach is quick, easy, and among the most flavorful recipes in the book. Fresh spinach, fresh garlic, a little broth, oil, salt, and pepper—and it's ready.

Carrots in Garlic Sauce is also quick and can be made in advance and heated right before serving. Following the *plain entree/fancy vegetable* rule, prepare Mustard-Cream Broccoli and Carrots, Creamed Spinach "Soufflé," or Swiss Chard Fritters to accompany a piece of poached chicken or fish or a slice of lean meat. Or try some of our simple vegetable dishes such as Lemon Broccoli, Braised Fresh Tomatoes, or Julienne of Carrots and Turnips.

For a low-fat Saint Patrick's Day dinner, buy lean slices of corned beef (or turkey pastrami) from your local deli and serve the meat with Buttered Cabbage and Potatoes. Roast your holiday turkey and surprise your guests with Sweet Potato Soufflé with Cranberry–Grand Marnier Coulis instead of canned yams and marshmallows.

You will find that you can mix and match all the green leafy vegetables in this chapter.

COOKING METHODS

Peeling and Seeding Tomatoes

To peel and seed fresh tomatoes, immerse them in boiling water for 30 seconds. Immediately plunge them into cold water, then peel the skins—they will literally fall away from the sides. Cut the skinned tomatoes in half horizontally, then squeeze out the seeds, reserving the liquid. The tomatoes are now ready to chop.

Steaming

Invest in a collapsible metal steamer if you don't already have one. They are inexpensive, easy to store, and a foolproof method to cook most vegetables to perfection. Steaming also locks in vitamins. To steam vegetables, place the steamer in a large pan with about an inch of water and bring the water to a boil. Place the vegetables in the steamer basket and cover the pan with a tightly fitting lid. Reduce the heat to medium; the water should stay lightly boiling. (Don't lift the lid until the vegetables are done.)

Cooking time depends on the size and thickness of the vegetables. Leafy greens, such as spinach, kale, Swiss chard, and turnip greens, should cook 1 to 2 minutes if the leaves are left whole. Cabbage quarters, whole carrots (unpeeled and scrubbed), brussels sprouts, broccoli with stalks, and large chunks of squash take 15 to 25 minutes, depending on their size. Rutabagas (cut into large chunks), whole new potatoes, and whole cauliflower cook in 20 to 30 minutes. Serve steamed vegetables with just a sprinkling of fresh lemon juice or chopped parsley to accompany a rich entree.

Stir-Frying

Stir-fried vegetables retain almost all of their vitamin content, and they remain crisp yet tender when cooked by this method. To stir-fry, heat a wok or large metal pan over high heat. When the metal is hot enough to make a drop of water sizzle, coat the pan with a minimal amount of corn oil or peanut oil—both are good for high-heat cooking. (Don't use olive oil; it will smoke and burn.) Add the vegetables and cook them on high until they're tender. Cooking time will be a matter of minutes. The curved sides of the wok make it easy to rotate vegetables so they will cook evenly.

You can also turn stir-fried vegetables into a meal by adding small strips of lean beef, pieces of poultry or fish, or cubed tofu flavored with soy sauce. Almost all vegetables can be stir-fried. Steam thick or dense vegetables such as turnips and cauliflower before stir-frying them to minimize cooking time needed in the wok. When stir-frying combinations, cook the thicker vegetables first, adding the thinner, faster-cooking ones last. Simple stir-fried vegetables are appropriate with any entree, plain or fancy.

A Few Don'ts

- Don't cook vegetables in an excessive amount of water—they lose vitamins and become soggy.
- Don't overcook vegetables—they lose flavor, texture, and some vitamins.
- Don't overseason; you want to taste the vegetable, not the spices.

BRAISED FRESH TOMATOES

*A variation of a classic garnish, these flavorful tomatoes can be used
as a vegetable or as an accompaniment to many of our vegetarian entrees.
If you don't have homegrown, use roma tomatoes.*

Makes 8 servings

1 tablespoon butter

½ cup sliced scallion

1⅓ cups chopped yellow
  onion

3 pounds tomatoes, peeled,
  seeded, and diced

6 cloves garlic, minced

3 bay leaves

½ teaspoon salt

¼ teaspoon dried thyme

¼ teaspoon pepper

Heat the butter in a heavy skillet until it's foamy. Add the scallion and onion
and sauté the vegetables until the onion is transparent. Add the remaining
ingredients and simmer the tomatoes, covered, for 30 minutes.

Braised tomatoes may be served chilled, at room temperature, or heated. They
will keep covered in the refrigerator for a few days.

Nutritional Analysis

Per Serving

Calories (kcal)	62.5	Cholesterol (mg)	4.0
Total Fat (g)	2.0	Dietary Fiber (g)	2.6
Saturated Fat (g)	1.0	% Calories from Fat	26.0
Monounsaturated Fat (g)	0.5	Vitamin C (mg)	35.0
Polyunsaturated Fat (g)	0.3	Vitamin A (i.u.)	1,086.0

Braised Leeks and Carrots

Braising is a wonderful technique for slowly cooking vegetables at low heat to allow the flavors to develop.

Makes 6 servings

6 small leeks (about 1 pound)

6 medium carrots (about 1 pound)

2 cups low-fat chicken broth

6 cloves garlic, split

2 tablespoons fresh lemon juice

1 teaspoon dried oregano

½ teaspoon dried thyme

½ teaspoon white pepper

Preheat the oven to 300°F.

Trim the leek root hairs to be even with the base (don't cut the base, as it holds the leeks together during cooking). Cut the leeks to a length of 6 inches from the root. Then cut them in half lengthwise (through the root) and wash them gently. Also trim the carrots to a length of 6 inches and cut them in half lengthwise.

Bring 3 cups water to a boil in a medium-size saucepan and add the leeks. Simmer the leeks for 5 minutes, or until they're barely fork-tender. Remove the leeks from the water and set them aside. Bring the water to a boil again (change the water if it's cloudy) and add the carrots. Simmer the carrots for 8 minutes, or until they're barely fork-tender. Remove the carrots from the pot and discard the water. Arrange the leeks and carrots in an attractive pattern in an ovenproof serving dish.

Combine the broth and the remaining ingredients and pour the mixture over the vegetables. Bake for 30 minutes.

Serve this course "family style" straight from the oven, or dish it up onto plates. Perfect as a hot vegetable or as a chilled salad.

Nutritional Analysis

Per Serving

Calories (kcal)	73.6	Cholesterol (mg)	0.0
Total Fat (g)	0.3	Dietary Fiber (g)	3.0
Saturated Fat (g)	0.0	% Calories from Fat	3.2
Monounsaturated Fat (g)	0.0	Vitamin C (mg)	16.0
Polyunsaturated Fat (g)	0.2	Vitamin A (i.u.)	18,099.0

Broccoli and Red Pepper Ragout

This is a lovely holiday dish with the brightness of the red peppers and broccoli. The dressing is light and allows the wonderful flavor of the vegetables to come through.

Makes 12 servings

4 pounds broccoli	6 tablespoons fresh lemon juice
1 pound red bell peppers	½ teaspoon garlic powder
½ cup low-fat chicken broth	½ teaspoon salt
1 tablespoon olive oil	½ teaspoon white pepper

Remove the stems from the broccoli. Cut off the ends and peel the stems with a paring knife. Slice the stems into ½-inch pieces. Cut the florets into even-size pieces. Steam the sliced stems for 5 minutes. Add the florets and steam 5 minutes more, until the florets and stems are barely fork-tender. Remove the broccoli from the heat immediately and quickly immerse it in cold water to halt the cooking process. Drain it well and allow it to cool.

Slice the peppers in half crosswise, remove the seeds and ribs, and slice the meat into strips. Steam the peppers for 1 to 2 minutes, until they're barely fork-tender. Drain the peppers and let them cool.

Mix the broth and remaining ingredients in a blender or whisk them together well. Toss the broccoli and peppers with the dressing. Marinate the vegetables in the dressing for several hours, or overnight, in the refrigerator.

Serve the ragout at room temperature (the flavor comes through better than when food is cold).

Nutritional Analysis

Per Serving

Calories (kcal)	65.8	Cholesterol (mg)	0.0
Total Fat (g)	1.7	Dietary Fiber (g)	5.4
Saturated Fat (g)	0.2	% Calories from Fat	18.9
Monounsaturated Fat (g)	0.9	Vitamin C (mg)	178.0
Polyunsaturated Fat (g)	0.4	Vitamin A (i.u.)	2,573.0

Buttered Cabbage and Potatoes

Known in Irish cuisine as colcannon, this simple country mainstay sometimes squeaks as it cooks.

Makes 6 servings

4 medium potatoes (about 1¼ pounds)

1 pound cabbage, chopped coarse

2 tablespoons butter

1 cup sliced scallion

¾ cup low-fat (1%) milk

1 teaspoon dried thyme

½ teaspoon salt

¼ teaspoon white pepper

Peel the potatoes, cut them into cubes, and boil them gently in a large pot of water until they're tender, about 10 minutes. Drain the potatoes well and gently mash them with a fork. Set the mashed potatoes aside.

Steam (or boil) the cabbage for about 8 minutes, just until tender. Set it aside.

In a large frying pan, heat the butter over medium-low heat until it's foamy. Add the scallion and sauté it until softened, about 3 minutes. Add the mashed potatoes and stir the vegetables to combine them. Add the milk, reduce the heat to low, and gently stir the mixture until the milk is incorporated into the potatoes and scallion. Add the cabbage, thyme, salt, and pepper and cook the mixture over low heat, stirring constantly, until all the ingredients are heated through.

Serve hot.

Nutritional Analysis

Per Serving

Calories (kcal)	209.6	Cholesterol (mg)	14.0
Total Fat (g)	5.1	Dietary Fiber (g)	3.9
Saturated Fat (g)	3.1	% Calories from Fat	21.3
Monounsaturated Fat (g)	1.4	Vitamin C (mg)	59.0
Polyunsaturated Fat (g)	0.3	Vitamin A (i.u.)	331.0

Cajun Greens and Turnips

This Cajun treat uses mustard greens. You can easily substitute spinach or kale.

Makes 6 servings

½ pound mustard greens

3 medium turnips

2 teaspoons olive oil

1 tablespoon low-fat chicken broth

1 cup chopped yellow onion

½ teaspoon sugar

½ teaspoon salt

⅛ teaspoon cayenne

Wash the greens and coarsely chop them. Steam them until they're just wilted, then drain them. Chop the turnips into ½-inch pieces and steam them just until they're fork-tender, and drain.

Heat the oil and broth together in a large skillet, add the onion, and sauté it until it's soft. Add the turnips, greens, sugar, salt, and cayenne to the onion mixture and heat it through, tossing the ingredients to combine them well.

Serve hot.

Nutritional Analysis

Per Serving

Calories (kcal)	48.3	Cholesterol (mg)	0.0
Total Fat (g)	1.7	Dietary Fiber (g)	2.1
Saturated Fat (g)	0.2	% Calories from Fat	28.3
Monounsaturated Fat (g)	1.1	Vitamin C (mg)	37.0
Polyunsaturated Fat (g)	0.2	Vitamin A (i.u.)	1,880.0

Carrots in Garlic Sauce

Besides being colorful, with the bright orange carrots and green flecks of fresh parsley, this dish can be quickly prepared even a day ahead and placed in the oven 20 minutes before dinner. It contains 385 percent of the amount of vitamin A (beta-carotene) you need daily.

Makes 6 servings

1 pound carrots, unpeeled, scrubbed, and sliced

3 cloves garlic, quartered

1 teaspoon chilled butter

¼ cup low-fat chicken broth

½ cup finely chopped fresh parsley

Preheat the oven to 350°F.

Steam the carrots for about 5 minutes, until they're just tender. Drain them and arrange them in a shallow baking dish. Bury the garlic quarters in among the carrot slices, distributing them evenly. Cut the butter into several pieces and place them over the carrot slices. Pour the broth on top.

Bake the carrots, covered, for 20 minutes, or until tender throughout.

Remove the garlic, if you like, and stir the dish. Sprinkle the carrots with the parsley, and serve.

Nutritional Analysis

Per Serving

Calories (kcal)	39.0	Cholesterol (mg)	2.0
Total Fat (g)	0.8	Dietary Fiber (g)	2.2
Saturated Fat (g)	0.4	% Calories from Fat	16.4
Monounsaturated Fat (g)	0.2	Vitamin C (mg)	13.0
Polyunsaturated Fat (g)	0.1	Vitamin A (i.u.)	19,227.0

Creamed Spinach "Soufflé"

This dish is loaded with beta-carotene and vitamin C.

Makes 4 servings

10 ounces frozen chopped
spinach

1 egg, beaten

2 teaspoons olive oil

1 tablespoon low-fat chicken
broth

½ cup sliced scallion

2 cloves garlic, minced

½ cup chopped mushrooms

½ cup grated carrot

2 tablespoons flour

¾ cup evaporated skim milk

½ teaspoon salt

¼ teaspoon pepper

⅛ teaspoon nutmeg

Preheat the oven to 350°F. Coat a standard-size (9" × 5" × 3") loaf pan with cooking spray.

Defrost the spinach and squeeze it dry. Using a fork, mix the spinach thoroughly with the egg until the mixture is light and fluffy.

Heat the oil and broth in a skillet over medium heat. Add the scallion and garlic and sauté until the scallion is softened but not browned. Add the mushrooms and carrot, reduce the heat to medium-low, and cook the vegetables for about 5 minutes, or until the liquid is evaporated. Add the flour and stir the pan to coat the vegetables. Add the milk and bring the contents to a boil, stirring. Reduce the heat and continue to stir for 2 to 3 minutes, until the mixture is thickened.

Remove the pan from the heat and stir in the egg-spinach mixture. Season the batter with the salt, pepper, and nutmeg and transfer it to the loaf pan. Bake the "soufflé" for 25 minutes, or until the center is firm.

Cut the loaf into slices and serve hot, or refrigerate it and serve chilled portions for a lighter meal.

Nutritional Analysis

Per Serving

Calories (kcal)	118.3	Cholesterol (mg)	47.0
Total Fat (g)	3.8	Dietary Fiber (g)	3.1
Saturated Fat (g)	0.8	% Calories from Fat	27.2
Monounsaturated Fat (g)	2.1	Vitamin C (mg)	25.0
Polyunsaturated Fat (g)	0.5	Vitamin A (i.u.)	9,240.0

Garlic-Sautéed Spinach

This recipe is simple and quick to make and allows the wonderful combination of flavors from the olive oil, garlic, and broth to merge into a great way to enjoy spinach.

Makes 4 servings

1 teaspoon olive oil

2 tablespoons low-fat chicken broth

3 cloves garlic, minced

2 pounds spinach, freshly washed and squeezed dry

½ teaspoon salt

¼ teaspoon pepper

Heat the oil and broth together in a large skillet over medium heat. Add the garlic and cook the mixture for 2 minutes. Raise the heat to medium-high, add the spinach, and sauté it just until the leaves are limp, tossing constantly with two large spoons.

Season the dish with the salt and pepper and serve immediately.

Nutritional Analysis

Per Serving

Calories (kcal)	49.7	Cholesterol (mg)	0.0
Total Fat (g)	1.7	Dietary Fiber (g)	4.5
Saturated Fat (g)	0.2	% Calories from Fat	24.7
Monounsaturated Fat (g)	0.8	Vitamin C (mg)	47.0
Polyunsaturated Fat (g)	0.3	Vitamin A (i.u.)	1,097.0

Julienne of Carrots and Turnips

This is a true "winter" vegetable dish, high in beta-carotene and vitamin C. Its versatility makes it perfect for holiday turkeys.

Makes 6 servings

1 pound carrots, peeled

1 pound turnips or rutabagas

2 teaspoons butter

2 tablespoons low-fat chicken broth

½ teaspoon salt

¼ teaspoon pepper

¼ teaspoon dried thyme

Cut the carrots and turnips into 2-inch pieces, then cut each piece into matchstick-size pieces, known as julienne-cut. Steam the vegetables until they're just tender, about 3 minutes. Drain them well. The vegetables may be done ahead and refrigerated at this point.

Just before serving, melt the butter with the broth in a skillet over medium-high heat. Toss the vegetables gently in the butter-broth mixture to coat them well. Season the julienne with the salt, pepper, and thyme. Heat the vegetables thoroughly but do not overcook them.

Nutritional Analysis

Per Serving

Calories (kcal)	57.4	Cholesterol (mg)	3.0
Total Fat (g)	1.4	Dietary Fiber (g)	3.2
Saturated Fat (g)	0.8	% Calories from Fat	20.9
Monounsaturated Fat (g)	0.4	Vitamin C (mg)	19.0
Polyunsaturated Fat (g)	0.1	Vitamin A (i.u.)	18,993.0

LEMON BROCCOLI

*This vitamin C–rich dish is another one that can be prepared ahead and baked
at the last minute. Great for busy nights or entertaining. The garlic
and fresh lemon juice are naturals with this bright green vegetable.*

Makes 6 servings

2 pounds broccoli

½ cup dry unseasoned bread
    crumbs

1 teaspoon lemon zest

1 tablespoon olive oil

2 cloves garlic, minced

¼ cup low-fat chicken broth

1 tablespoon fresh lemon juice

½ teaspoon salt

¼ teaspoon pepper

Preheat the oven to 300°F.

Break the broccoli into florets. Cut the ends off of the stems and peel the
outside of the stalks with a paring knife. Slice the tender inside of the stalks
and place them in a steamer with the florets. Steam the broccoli until almost
tender.

In a nonstick skillet, heat the bread crumbs over very low heat, stirring often,
until they turn a golden color. Remove the crumbs from the skillet and mix
them with the lemon zest. Set the crumb mixture aside.

In the same skillet, heat the oil over medium-low heat, add the garlic, and
sauté it until it's light golden (don't allow the garlic to brown—it makes the
garlic bitter). Add the broth, lemon juice, salt, and pepper. Toss the broccoli
gently in the broth mixture to coat it evenly. Transfer the contents to a baking
dish and top the broccoli with the lemon-crumbs. Bake for 5 to 10 minutes, or
until the broccoli and sauce are hot. Don't overcook.

Nutritional Analysis

Per Serving

Calories (kcal)	101.8	Cholesterol (mg)	0.0
Total Fat (g)	3.4	Dietary Fiber (g)	5.1
Saturated Fat (g)	0.5	% Calories from Fat	26.1
Monounsaturated Fat (g)	2.0	Vitamin C (mg)	143.0
Polyunsaturated Fat (g)	0.5	Vitamin A (i.u.)	2,334.0

Mustard-Cream Broccoli and Carrots

This is a great dish for a buffet dinner, as it can be completely prepared ahead and served at room temperature. It is delicious, extremely healthful, and certainly elegant. For an extra-special touch, sprinkle chopped fresh chives and lemon zest on top. This recipe is low in both calories and percentage of calories from fat.

Makes 6 servings

1 pound carrots, unpeeled and scrubbed

2 cups low-fat chicken broth

1 pound broccoli stalks

3 tablespoons low-fat yogurt

2 tablespoons chopped watercress

2 tablespoons sliced scallion

1 teaspoon Dijon mustard

1 teaspoon fresh lemon juice

½ teaspoon salt

½ teaspoon sugar

¼ teaspoon pepper

Cut the carrots into long sticks. Heat the broth to a boil, add the carrots, and simmer them for 5 minutes. Remove the carrots with a slotted spoon, leaving the broth in the pan.

Peel the outer tough skin off the broccoli stalks and cut the inside into long sticks about the same size as the carrot sticks. Bring the broth used to cook the carrots to a boil again, add the broccoli, and simmer for 3 minutes. Drain the broccoli, again saving the broth. Keep the vegetables separate.

Combine 3 tablespoons of the broth used to cook the vegetables with the remaining ingredients to make the sauce. Divide the sauce in half and marinate the vegetables in separate bowls for several hours.

Serve the vegetables chilled or at room temperature in the marinade, alongside one another.

Nutritional Analysis

Per Serving

Calories (kcal)	55.9	Cholesterol (mg)	0.0
Total Fat (g)	0.4	Dietary Fiber (g)	2.1
Saturated Fat (g)	0.1	% Calories from Fat	5.2
Monounsaturated Fat (g)	0.1	Vitamin C (mg)	51.0
Polyunsaturated Fat (g)	0.1	Vitamin A (i.u.)	19,171.0

Oven-Roasted Vegetables

These vegetables are great alone but have a lot of other uses as well. Try them on French bread for a roasted vegetable sandwich; toss them with pasta and a bit of olive oil and sprinkle the mix with a bit of fresh Asiago cheese; or make a marinated vegetable salad by drizzling them with some balsamic vinegar.

Makes 8 servings

24 2-inch sliced asparagus spears

8 cloves garlic, halved

2 medium zucchini, cut into 1-inch slices

2 medium yellow squash, cut into 1-inch slices

1 medium red bell pepper, cut into 1-inch cubes

1 medium yellow bell pepper, cut into 1-inch cubes

1 medium green bell pepper, cut into 1-inch cubes

1 tablespoon olive oil

½ cup chopped fresh Italian parsley

¼ cup chopped fresh basil

½ teaspoon salt

½ teaspoon ground black pepper

Preheat the oven to 425°F.

Coat a large baking sheet with cooking spray.

Combine the vegetables in a large bowl and drizzle them with the oil. Toss to coat the vegetables well. Add the parsley, basil, salt, and black pepper and toss again to coat all the vegetables evenly.

Place the vegetables in a single layer on the baking sheet and bake them for 15 minutes; turn the vegetables and bake for 5 minutes longer.

Serve the dish warm or at room temperature.

Nutritional Analysis

Per Serving

Calories (kcal)	60.3	Cholesterol (mg)	0.0
Total Fat (g)	2.1	Dietary Fiber (g)	3.8
Saturated Fat (g)	0.3	% Calories from Fat	26.4
Monounsaturated Fat (g)	1.3	Vitamin C (mg)	52.0
Polyunsaturated Fat (g)	0.3	Vitamin A (i.u.)	1,590.0

South American Carrots

This recipe is based on a traditional South American dish called "carrot farofa."
It is delicious and beautifully colored. If you're serving this course with food
that doesn't complement cilantro, use parsley, basil, or any fresh herb
of your choice instead of the cilantro leaves.

Makes 6 servings

1 teaspoon butter

1 teaspoon olive oil

3 tablespoons low-fat chicken broth

6 medium carrots, grated

⅓ cup dry unseasoned bread crumbs

½ teaspoon salt

¼ teaspoon white pepper

⅓ cup fresh cilantro leaves

Melt the butter with the oil and broth in a heavy skillet over medium heat. Add the carrots and sauté them for 5 minutes, or until they're tender. Add the bread crumbs, salt, and pepper and cook the mixture for 5 minutes longer.

Serve the carrots hot, sprinkled with the cilantro leaves.

Nutritional Analysis

Per Serving

Calories (kcal)	65.2	Cholesterol (mg)	2.0
Total Fat (g)	1.9	Dietary Fiber (g)	2.3
Saturated Fat (g)	0.6	% Calories from Fat	25.0
Monounsaturated Fat (g)	0.9	Vitamin C (mg)	6.0
Polyunsaturated Fat (g)	0.2	Vitamin A (i.u.)	18,071.0

SWEET POTATO SOUFFLÉ WITH CRANBERRY–GRAND MARNIER COULIS

This dish is elegant, and stunning with its brilliant fall colors.

Makes 6 servings

1 pound sweet potatoes, peeled and cubed	1 12-ounce bag fresh cranberries, additional
1 egg plus 2 egg whites	2 cups sugar
1 cup milk	⅔ cup Madeira
½ teaspoon salt	6 tablespoons Grand Marnier
½ cup cranberries	

Sweet Potato Soufflé

Preheat the oven to 350°F. Coat a 2-quart baking dish with cooking spray.

Steam or boil the sweet potatoes until they're tender. Drain the potatoes and allow them to cool. In a food processor or blender, combine the egg and egg whites, milk, and salt, and process the mixture until it's blended. Add the sweet potatoes and process until smooth. Add ½ cup of the cranberries and process the mixture until the berries are coarsely chopped.

Spread the sweet potato mixture in the baking dish and cover the dish with a sheet of foil. Set the dish in a pan large enough to accommodate it, and add 1 inch of boiling water to the pan. Bake for 1 hour to 1 hour and 15 minutes, until a knife inserted in the center comes out clean.

Grand Marnier Sauce

While the soufflé is baking, prepare the sauce by combining the 12-ounce bag of cranberries, the sugar, Madeira, and Grand Marnier. Bring the mixture to a boil, reduce the heat to medium-low, and simmer for 30 minutes. Puree the mixture, then strain it through a mesh strainer, pressing hard to extract as much fruit as possible, leaving the skins behind.

Serve the sauce over the warm soufflé.

Nutritional Analysis

Per Serving

Calories (kcal)	469.5	Cholesterol (mg)	36.0
Total Fat (g)	2.4	Dietary Fiber (g)	4.3
Saturated Fat (g)	1.1	% Calories from Fat	5.0
Monounsaturated Fat (g)	0.7	Vitamin C (mg)	21.0
Polyunsaturated Fat (g)	0.3	Vitamin A (i.u.)	11,055.0

Swiss Chard Fritters

This is a tasty use of vitamin-rich Swiss chard.

Makes 6 servings

1 cup flour

⅔ cup low-fat (1%) milk

2 eggs, beaten

1 tablespoon butter, melted and cooled

1 medium yellow onion, chopped fine

½ teaspoon salt

¼ teaspoon pepper

2 cups chopped Swiss chard leaves

Preheat the oven to 250°F.

In a large bowl, whisk the flour, milk, eggs, and butter to combine them. Add the onion, salt, and pepper and stir the mixture to blend the ingredients well. Fold in the Swiss chard until the leaves are well mixed.

Lightly coat a skillet or griddle with cooking spray and heat it to medium-hot. Use 2 tablespoons of batter for each fritter, pressing down on each mound to flatten it. Fry the fritters on each side until they're golden and slightly crisp. Repeat until all the batter is used, adding cooking spray to the pan as needed.

Keep the cooked fritters warm in a covered baking dish in the oven until you're ready to serve them.

Nutritional Analysis

Per Serving

Calories (kcal)	149.6	Cholesterol (mg)	67.0
Total Fat (g)	4.0	Dietary Fiber (g)	2.3
Saturated Fat (g)	1.8	% Calories from Fat	23.7
Monounsaturated Fat (g)	1.2	Vitamin C (mg)	26.0
Polyunsaturated Fat (g)	0.4	Vitamin A (i.u.)	2,820.0

White Beans with Garlic

These beans are delicious and can be served either warm or chilled.

Makes 8 servings

1 pound white beans	1 teaspoon dried basil
½ teaspoon salt	1 bunch fresh watercress,
¼ teaspoon pepper	chopped
2 cloves garlic, minced	2 tablespoons olive oil

Cover the beans with water in a saucepan and soak them for 8 to 12 hours. Drain the beans, cover them again with water, and bring them to a boil. Cover the pan and simmer the beans for 50 to 60 minutes, or until they're tender (don't overcook). Drain the beans and toss them gently with the salt, pepper, garlic, basil, watercress, and oil.

White beans may be served hot or as a chilled bean salad.

Nutritional Analysis

Per Serving

Calories (kcal)	220.8	Cholesterol (mg)	0.0
Total Fat (g)	3.9	Dietary Fiber (g)	8.8
Saturated Fat (g)	0.6	% Calories from Fat	15.3
Monounsaturated Fat (g)	2.5	Vitamin C (mg)	2.0
Polyunsaturated Fat (g)	0.5	Vitamin A (i.u.)	200.0

Winter Vegetables with Garlic and Herbs

The butter melts into the potatoes (using only 2 tablespoons for eight servings) and infuses the whole dish with a rich, flavorful taste without a high fat content.

Makes 8 servings

6 medium red potatoes, cubed

6 medium carrots, sliced

12 ounces fresh or frozen brussels sprouts

2 tablespoons butter

2 cloves garlic, minced

¼ cup sliced scallion

½ teaspoon dried thyme

½ teaspoon dried sage

½ teaspoon salt

¼ teaspoon pepper

¼ cup chopped fresh parsley

In a large saucepan, steam the potatoes and carrots for 10 minutes. Cut the sprouts in half, add them to the potatoes and carrots, and steam the vegetables for 10 minutes more, or until they're fork-tender (don't overcook).

Melt the butter in a large skillet. Add the garlic, scallion, thyme, sage, salt, and pepper and sauté for 5 minutes. Add the vegetables to the butter mixture and gently toss them, heating the vegetables thoroughly.

Sprinkle with the parsley and serve.

Nutritional Analysis

Per Serving

Calories (kcal)	115.2	Cholesterol (mg)	8.0
Total Fat (g)	3.2	Dietary Fiber (g)	4.2
Saturated Fat (g)	1.8	% Calories from Fat	23.5
Monounsaturated Fat (g)	0.9	Vitamin C (mg)	45.0
Polyunsaturated Fat (g)	0.2	Vitamin A (i.u.)	14,079.0

Grains,
Potatoes, and
Pasta

7

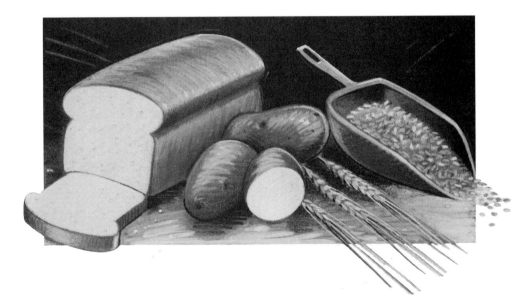

Pasta, grains, and potatoes, the darlings of the late '80s and '90s and the base for the USDA Food Pyramid, are suddenly getting a bad reputation. Why? They are low in fat and usually a good source of fiber. There is one simple reason—our portion sizes of these foods are much too big. Carbohydrates certainly have a place in a cancer risk-reduction eating plan, but we consume too much in a "serving size." Many nutritionists blame the excessive consumption of carbohydrates (while eschewing animal protein sources) for the shocking new statistics on obesity in America. The fact that these foods do not contain fat doesn't mean they are not fattening. Many restaurants now serve sauce-laden pasta on plates the size of serving platters. Baked potatoes in elegant steak houses are the size of small melons.

The American Cancer Society strongly recommends that we eat more whole grains. Whole grains are an important source of dietary fiber, trace minerals, vitamins, and other compounds that have been shown to be effective on a cancer risk-reduction diet, especially when combined with a diet high in fruits and vegetables. All of these compounds work synergistically. This is why we emphasize that vitamin supplements or fiber powders are *not* recommended. This chapter provides you with some wonderful recipes and a variety of uses for whole wheat, cornmeal, brown rice, barley, and potatoes.

Whole foods are best. By this we mean food in an unprocessed state. Over the years, in the name of progress, manufacturers have bleached, refined, and stripped grains so they will look prettier and have a softer texture. But in exchange, the foods have been depleted of their original nutrients.

Many people already use only 100 percent whole wheat products—flour, premade pasta, and noodles. The taste and texture of these products are quite different from "regular" flour and pastas. Admittedly they are an acquired taste when you switch from one product to another. Our recipes list the regular white pasta in the ingredients. However, all recipes were tested with whole wheat pasta and noodles, as well as a mixture of half-and-half.

To gradually introduce whole wheat pasta into your meals, start with one-quarter whole wheat and three-quarters white pasta or noodles. Increase the whole wheat products gradually to your own taste. This increases vitamin content and dietary fiber.

Whole wheat pastas and noodles are available in most supermarkets. Also try local health food stores. As for "vegetable" pastas such as spinach or beet, it has been our experience that a minimum amount of the vegetable has been added simply for color. Read the package: if the vegetable is at the end of the ingredients list, it is merely a food dye—certainly harmless, but containing only trace amounts of vitamins.

Chilled Chinese Noodles with Sesame Oil and Orange can be made with buckwheat noodles found in the Asian section of supermarkets or in Asian grocery stores.

Rice, another excellent grain, is probably the most universal food. Every country has its favorite rice dish. It is usually one of the first foods (in the form of infant rice cereal) that we give to babies. Steamed rice, baked rice, fried rice, or herbed rice—it is a food that is versatile, easy to cook, and suitable for any occasion. Rice comes in four forms: brown or whole, white (polished), parboiled or converted, and wild. Brown rice retains all the original nutrients of the rice kernel. White or polished rice is stripped of its outer layers and many of its vitamins, minerals, and fiber and some protein. Parboiled or converted rice retains more of the original nutrients because the process of parboiling pushes some of the vitamins from the bran to the white endosperm. Wild rice retains more nutrients and contains more fiber than white rice. It is used in recipes mostly for its texture and appearance. Although it is not interchangeable with white, it can be mixed with white rice as a nice alternative.

Brown rice versus white rice—which is better? Brown rice does contain more fiber, vitamins, and minerals than white rice. Nutritionally, brown rice wins right there. It also has a thicker consistency and crunchier texture than white rice, which make it a welcome addition to many vegetarian dishes. The taste is delicious, and you feel you are eating real substance. However, in some dishes, white rice is more aesthetically pleasing to the eye than natural brown rice. Note that some of the dishes using brown rice can be made with white rice, and vice versa. Just be sure to change the cooking time: brown rice takes longer to cook (see "Cooking Methods"). If the recipe calls for brown rice and you use white, the fiber per serving will be less than the value given for that recipe. Both Chicken Fried Rice and Vermicelli-Rice Pilaf are scrumptious, hearty, and filling.

We love potatoes! Both white and sweet potatoes rank high on a cancer risk-reduction eating plan. White potatoes contain vitamin C and are a good source of fiber with the skins left on. Sweet potatoes are extremely high in beta-carotene; one potato will supply you with almost twice the recommended daily requirement of vitamin A (beta-carotene). In this chapter we include some low-fat variations of high-fat favorites. Oven French Fries, Sweet Potato Fries, Scalloped Potatoes and Carrots, and Cheese-Stuffed Potatoes are just a few of these selections. Here again, this is a chapter where you pair a plain entree and a fancy side dish. Serve sliced turkey with Wild Rice with Dried Cranberries and Balsamic Vinegar; steamed baby carrots or broccoli completes this quick and lovely meal. Bake white fish in foil to keep it moist and serve it with Scalloped Potatoes and Carrots as accompaniment.

Cooking Methods

Brown Rice

Place 1¾ cups cold water and 1 cup rice in a saucepan. Cover the pan tightly and bring the water to a boil. Reduce the heat to low and simmer the rice for 40 minutes. Fluff the cooked rice with a fork. Yields about 3 cups.

White Rice

Follow the directions for brown rice, except use 1½ cups water and simmer white rice for only 20 minutes. Yields about 3 cups.

Cooking Perfect Pasta

Bring slightly salted water to a rapid boil in a large pot over high heat (the water will take about 10 minutes to reach a rapid boil). Add a few drops of olive oil to help prevent the pasta from sticking and to prevent the water from foaming over. Add the pasta a little at a time. When all the pasta is in the pot, stir it with a fork to separate it, and return the water to a boil. Stir the pot often to make sure the pasta doesn't stick together. Cooking time will depend on the size and thickness of the pasta. Thin pasta like vermicelli needs to boil for about 5 minutes. Thicker pasta like shells, 8 to 10 minutes.

Pasta should be cooked al dente—slightly chewy. To test for doneness, let a piece cool, and pinch or bite it. The pasta should be slightly resistant, yet flexible. Drain the pasta in a large colander, briskly shaking it to eliminate all excess moisture. It is important that the pasta be as dry as possible before you top it with sauce. Water seeping out from the edges of the pasta and diluting the sauce ruins a pasta dish.

An easy way to reheat leftover plain pasta (in case you cooked too much): Heat a large pot of water to rapid boiling. Put the pasta in a metal sieve. Dunk the sieve into the water for about 10 seconds and then drain the pasta. It will be warmed but not mushy from overcooking.

GRAINS

BARLEY PILAF

This pilaf is a tasty alternative to ordinary rice and grain dishes. The flecks of green from the scallion and parsley add color, while the cashews add an unexpected texture.

Makes 6 servings

1½ tablespoons butter

½ cup chopped scallion

1 cup rinsed and drained barley

2 cups low-fat chicken broth

½ teaspoon dried thyme

¼ teaspoon salt

¼ teaspoon white pepper

¼ cup dry-roasted and chopped cashews

¼ cup chopped fresh parsley

Heat the butter in a medium-size pan. When the butter starts to foam, add the scallion and sauté for 5 minutes. Add the barley, broth, thyme, salt, white pepper, and cashews. Bring the mixture to a boil, cover the pan, and simmer the contents for 40 to 50 minutes, or until the barley is tender.

Sprinkle the pilaf with the parsley before serving.

Nutritional Analysis

Per Serving

Calories (kcal)	176.5	Cholesterol (mg)	8.0
Total Fat (g)	6.2	Dietary Fiber (g)	5.2
Saturated Fat (g)	2.4	% Calories from Fat	28.9
Monounsaturated Fat (g)	2.5	Vitamin C (mg)	7.0
Polyunsaturated Fat (g)	0.9	Vitamin A (i.u.)	280.0

Chicken Fried Rice

This is a quick and easy dish, especially if you have leftover poultry, meat, or shellfish and some cooked rice. Use your imagination (or leftovers) and add whatever vegetables you happen to have on hand.

Makes 6 servings

1 cup uncooked brown rice

2 teaspoons canola oil

½ cup grated carrot

1 cup cooked and chopped
    chicken

2 eggs, slightly beaten

½ teaspoon pepper

3 tablespoons low-sodium soy
    sauce

⅔ cup sliced scallion

Begin cooking the rice according to the package directions, about 50 minutes before serving (if time is short, use white rice, as it cooks much faster).

Heat the oil in a large skillet over medium heat. Add the carrot and chicken and sauté for 1 minute, stirring constantly. Add the eggs and pepper and cook for 1 minute, stirring constantly. Add the rice and soy sauce and cook for 5 more minutes, tossing often to combine the ingredients well and prevent them from sticking.

Garnish the rice with the sliced scallion and serve.

Nutritional Analysis

Per Serving

Calories (kcal)	211.3	Cholesterol (mg)	81.0
Total Fat (g)	6.4	Dietary Fiber (g)	2.3
Saturated Fat (g)	1.4	% Calories from Fat	27.6
Monounsaturated Fat (g)	2.7	Vitamin C (mg)	6.0
Polyunsaturated Fat (g)	1.7	Vitamin A (i.u.)	2,433.0

PESTO AND SUN-DRIED TOMATO POLENTA

This dish may be served plain or with a tomato or meat sauce. Add a sprinkle of cheese, if you like. For a simple light meal, top polenta portions with leftover meat, fish, or poultry, spoon marinara sauce on top, and sprinkle each serving with a bit of freshly grated Asiago.

Makes 6 servings

1 cup polenta

3¼ cups lukewarm water

4 cloves garlic, minced

½ teaspoon salt

¼ teaspoon white pepper

3 tablespoons pesto sauce

3 tablespoons finely chopped sun-dried tomatoes

Preheat the oven to 350°F. Coat an 8-inch square pan with cooking spray.

Place the polenta, water, garlic, salt, and white pepper in the pan and stir the mixture with a fork until blended. Bake the polenta for 50 minutes, then stir in the pesto and sun-dried tomatoes with a fork and bake for 10 minutes more.

Serve the polenta directly from the oven or allow it to cool and cut into six pieces.

Nutritional Analysis

Per Serving

Calories (kcal)	129.4	Cholesterol (mg)	2.0
Total Fat (g)	4.0	Dietary Fiber (g)	2.0
Saturated Fat (g)	0.9	% Calories from Fat	27.5
Monounsaturated Fat (g)	2.3	Vitamin C (mg)	2.0
Polyunsaturated Fat (g)	0.4	Vitamin A (i.u.)	187.0

VERMICELLI-RICE PILAF

*This pilaf is much better than plain rice, and rather elegant—a good complement
to special entrees. The rich buttery flavor is a treat, wonderful to enjoy
on occasion—especially since the recipe has only 20.9 calories from fat!*

Makes 6 servings

2 tablespoons butter

½ cup vermicelli, broken into
   1-inch pieces

¼ cup sliced scallion

1 cup brown rice

½ teaspoon dried oregano

½ teaspoon celery salt

¼ teaspoon pepper

1½ cups low-fat chicken broth

Melt the butter in a saucepan over medium heat. When the butter starts to
foam, add the vermicelli and scallion and sauté for 5 minutes. Add the rice,
oregano, celery salt, pepper, and broth and bring the mixture to a boil. Stir
well, cover the pan, reduce the heat, and simmer the contents gently for
50 minutes.

Fluff the pilaf with a fork and serve.

Nutritional Analysis

Per Serving

Calories (kcal)	188.9	Cholesterol (mg)	10.0
Total Fat (g)	4.7	Dietary Fiber (g)	0.7
Saturated Fat (g)	2.5	% Calories from Fat	20.9
Monounsaturated Fat (g)	1.4	Vitamin C (mg)	2.0
Polyunsaturated Fat (g)	0.4	Vitamin A (i.u.)	168.0

Wild Rice–Cranberry Stuffing

*This tasty blend may be used as a stuffing for poultry or as a side dish.
It is unusual and delicious, with cranberry-studded wild and white rice.
(You can easily use brown rice instead, but be sure to adjust the cooking
time because brown rice takes longer to prepare.)*

Makes 8 servings

1½ quarts low-fat chicken
  broth

6 ounces wild rice

1 tablespoon butter

½ cup chopped mushrooms

½ cup chopped yellow onion

½ cup chopped carrot

½ cup chopped celery

1 cup white rice

1½ cups cranberries

1 teaspoon dried thyme

½ teaspoon white pepper

3 bay leaves

Bring 3 cups of the broth to a boil. Add the wild rice and boil, uncovered, for 40 minutes (add more water if necessary).

Melt the butter in a large pan. Add the mushrooms, onion, carrot, and celery and sauté the vegetables for 5 minutes. Add the white rice and sauté for 5 minutes. Add the cranberries and sauté for an additional 5 minutes. Add the remaining 3 cups broth, the cooked wild rice, thyme, pepper, and bay leaves. Bring the contents to a boil, reduce the heat, cover the pan, and simmer the mixture for 30 minutes, or until the liquid is absorbed.

Discard the bay leaves before serving.

Nutritional Analysis

Per Serving

Calories (kcal)	207.4	Cholesterol (mg)	4.0
Total Fat (g)	2.0	Dietary Fiber (g)	3.2
Saturated Fat (g)	1.0	% Calories from Fat	7.5
Monounsaturated Fat (g)	0.5	Vitamin C (mg)	5.0
Polyunsaturated Fat (g)	0.3	Vitamin A (i.u.)	1,845.0

Wild Rice with Dried Cranberries and Balsamic Vinegar

This is such an interesting dish, with the hearty wild rice complemented by the tang of the balsamic vinegar and slight sweetness from the dried cranberries. It has lots of flavor, especially for 2.6 percent calories from fat!

Makes 6 servings

6 ounces wild rice	¼ cup dried cranberries
¼ teaspoon salt	2 tablespoons balsamic vinegar
¼ teaspoon white pepper	

Rinse the rice thoroughly. Bring 2 quarts of water to a full boil and add the rice. Bring the water to a second boil and continue to cook the rice at a full boil for 50 minutes, or until tender. Drain, if necessary, and add the remaining ingredients.

May be served hot or chilled as a salad.

Nutritional Analysis

Per Serving

Calories (kcal)	106.5	Cholesterol (mg)	0.0
Total Fat (g)	0.3	Dietary Fiber (g)	2.1
Saturated Fat (g)	0.0	% Calories from Fat	2.6
Monounsaturated Fat (g)	0.3	Vitamin C (mg)	1.0
Polyunsaturated Fat (g)	0.2	Vitamin A (i.u.)	9.0

Potatoes

Cheese-Stuffed Potatoes

These may be made a day ahead. We usually serve them for the holidays,
to avoid last-minute mashing of potatoes.

Makes 6 servings

6 medium baking potatoes

1½ tablespoons butter, at room temperature

2 tablespoons low-fat chicken broth

¼ cup low-fat (1%) milk

¼ cup part-skim ricotta cheese

½ teaspoon salt

½ teaspoon white pepper

3 tablespoons dry unseasoned bread crumbs

6 tablespoons sliced scallion

Baked Potatoes

Preheat the oven to 375°F.

Bake the potatoes for 45 minutes to 1 hour, until tender. Remove the potatoes, but leave the oven on. Cut a lengthwise slice off the top of each potato and carefully scoop out most of the center, leaving enough to support the shell.

Stuffing

Mash the potato centers with a fork, then add the butter, broth, milk, ricotta, salt, and white pepper, mixing just until the ingredients are combined. Combine the bread crumbs and scallion. Fill the shells with the potato mixture and sprinkle each potato with the bread crumb mixture.

Return the stuffed potatoes to the oven and bake them for 25 minutes, or until they're heated through.

Nutritional Analysis

Per Serving

Calories (kcal)	149.1	Cholesterol (mg)	11.0
Total Fat (g)	4.1	Dietary Fiber (g)	2.1
Saturated Fat (g)	2.4	% Calories from Fat	24.1
Monounsaturated Fat (g)	1.2	Vitamin C (mg)	25.0
Polyunsaturated Fat (g)	0.2	Vitamin A (i.u.)	196.0

Garlic-Chive Mashed Potatoes

You're not likely to find tastier mashed potatoes than these; what you won't find is the high fat content that the dish usually contains. Not peeling the potatoes—and incorporating sautéed garlic and fresh chives—adds color, texture, fiber, and a superb flavor.

Makes 8 servings

2 heads garlic (about 30 cloves)

1 tablespoon butter

1 tablespoon olive oil

2 tablespoons flour

1¼ cups 2% milk

½ teaspoon salt

¼ teaspoon pepper

½ cup chopped fresh chives

2½ pounds potatoes, unpeeled and cut into 1-inch cubes

¼ cup minced fresh parsley

Separate the garlic heads into cloves and peel them. Heat the butter and oil in a large pan over low heat. Add the garlic and cook, covered, for 30 minutes, stirring occasionally to prevent burning. Add the flour, mixing well. Add 1 cup of the milk, the salt, and pepper and bring the mixture to a boil. Reduce the heat, add the chives, and stir for 2 minutes. Remove the pan from the heat and mash the contents with a potato masher (or use a food processor or blender). Cover the garlic mixture to keep it warm.

Meanwhile, boil the potatoes until they're tender. Drain the potatoes and mash them with a potato masher or fork (overmixing can make them gummy). Heat the remaining ¼ cup milk in a large saucepan and beat in the hot potatoes. Add the warm garlic mixture and mix gently but thoroughly.

Sprinkle the potatoes with the parsley and serve.

Nutritional Analysis

Per Serving

Calories (kcal)	144.8	Cholesterol (mg)	9.0
Total Fat (g)	4.6	Dietary Fiber (g)	1.9
Saturated Fat (g)	1.9	% Calories from Fat	27.7
Monounsaturated Fat (g)	2.0	Vitamin C (mg)	26.0
Polyunsaturated Fat (g)	0.3	Vitamin A (i.u.)	330.0

Oven French Fries

These aren't the traditional fat-laden french fries, but they are fabulous.

Makes 6 servings

2 pounds potatoes, unpeeled

1½ tablespoons canola oil

½ teaspoon salt

½ teaspoon pepper

½ teaspoon paprika

Preheat the oven to 375°F.

Cut the potatoes into large sticks. In a large bowl, toss the potato sticks with the oil to coat them thoroughly. Combine the salt, pepper, and paprika and sprinkle the mixture over the potatoes. Toss the potatoes again to distribute the spices. Place the potato sticks on a baking sheet (preferably a nonstick one) in a single layer. Bake the potatoes for 20 minutes; loosen them with a metal spatula and gently toss them, then bake for 20 minutes longer. Loosen the oven fries with a metal spatula and serve.

Nutritional Analysis

Per Serving

Calories (kcal)	120.7	Cholesterol (mg)	0.0
Total Fat (g)	3.5	Dietary Fiber (g)	1.9
Saturated Fat (g)	0.3	% Calories from Fat	25.7
Monounsaturated Fat (g)	2.1	Vitamin C (mg)	23.0
Polyunsaturated Fat (g)	1.1	Vitamin A (i.u.)	106.0

POTATO-CHEESE PANCAKES

These pancakes are delicious alone or served with nonfat yogurt.

Makes 8 servings

4 cups grated, unpeeled
  potatoes

½ teaspoon salt plus additional
  for seasoning the potatoes

6 ounces grated mozzarella
  cheese, part skim

2 cloves garlic, minced

4 eggs, beaten

2 cups grated carrot

⅔ cup flour

½ cup chopped fresh parsley

¼ cup minced yellow onion

2 tablespoons fresh lemon juice

½ teaspoon pepper

Lightly salt the potatoes and allow them to drain for 15 minutes. Squeeze the potatoes to get rid of excess water. Combine the potatoes with the remaining ingredients to make the batter.

Heat a nonstick pan, or one coated with cooking spray, to medium-high. Use approximately ¼ cup batter for each pancake, pressing down with a spatula to make the pancakes thin. Fry each cake for about 2 minutes per side, until browned and crisp. Keep the cooked pancakes warm while you fry the remainder by placing them in a single layer on a baking sheet in a warming oven.

Nutritional Analysis

Per Serving

Calories (kcal)	215.4	Cholesterol (mg)	103.0
Total Fat (g)	6.0	Dietary Fiber (g)	2.7
Saturated Fat (g)	3.0	% Calories from Fat	25.1
Monounsaturated Fat (g)	1.9	Vitamin C (mg)	27.0
Polyunsaturated Fat (g)	0.5	Vitamin A (i.u.)	7,344.0

SCALLION MASHED POTATOES

This recipe contains just enough butter to lend a delicious richness and flavor to the mashed potatoes without making them fat laden. The warm milk helps to achieve a light texture usually obtained solely from butter.

Makes 6 servings

2 pounds potatoes, peeled and
  quartered

4 scallions, sliced

¾ cup low-fat (1%) milk

½ teaspoon salt

½ teaspoon white pepper

2 tablespoons butter, at room
  temperature

Boil the potatoes until they're tender and drain them well.

While the potatoes are cooking, simmer the scallion in the milk for 5 minutes. Remove the milk mixture from the heat and cover the pan to keep it warm until the potatoes are done. Mash the potatoes while they are still hot, gradually adding the warm milk mixture. Add the salt, white pepper, and butter and mix just until the ingredients are combined (don't overbeat, or the potatoes will be heavy and gummy).

Serve hot.

Nutritional Analysis

Per Serving

Calories (kcal)	167.4	Cholesterol (mg)	11.0
Total Fat (g)	4.4	Dietary Fiber (g)	4.3
Saturated Fat (g)	2.6	% Calories from Fat	22.4
Monounsaturated Fat (g)	1.2	Vitamin C (mg)	66.0
Polyunsaturated Fat (g)	0.3	Vitamin A (i.u.)	577.0

SCALLOPED POTATOES AND CARROTS

The nonfat dry milk combined with the liquid milk adds a richness that is usually achieved by using cream. These potatoes are much lighter in fat than traditional scalloped potatoes and have an extra boost of calcium from the dry milk, as well as loads of vitamins C and A (beta-carotene).

Makes 6 servings

2 cups sliced carrot

½ teaspoon salt

½ cup sliced scallion

2 pounds potatoes, peeled and sliced thin

¼ teaspoon pepper

6 tablespoons grated Parmesan cheese

1½ tablespoons cold butter, cut in 9 pieces

1½ cups low-fat (1%) milk

5 tablespoons nonfat dry milk

Preheat the oven to 350°F. Coat a large casserole dish with cooking spray.

Steam the carrots until they're barely tender. Drain the carrots and toss them with ¼ teaspoon of the salt and the scallion.

Making three layers, arrange one-third of the potatoes, then one-third of the carrot mixture, seasoning each layer with some of the remaining ¼ teaspoon salt, the pepper, cheese, and pieces of butter. Repeat to make three layers. Whisk the 1% milk with the dry milk and pour the liquid over the vegetables.

Cover the casserole and bake it for 1 hour, then remove cover, baste the top with the liquid, and bake for 30 minutes longer.

Nutritional Analysis

Per Serving

Calories (kcal)	208.6	Cholesterol (mg)	16.0
Total Fat (g)	5.6	Dietary Fiber (g)	3.0
Saturated Fat (g)	3.4	% Calories from Fat	23.8
Monounsaturated Fat (g)	1.6	Vitamin C (mg)	30.0
Polyunsaturated Fat (g)	0.2	Vitamin A (i.u.)	9,484.0

Sweet Potato Fries

These fries are a colorful and delicious addition to meat, poultry, pork, fish, or veal. They hold their shape, but they will not be crispy. Sweet potatoes are a vegetable that ranks among the highest in beta-carotene content.

Makes 4 servings

1 pound sweet potatoes, unpeeled

1 tablespoon canola oil

½ teaspoon salt

Preheat the oven to 350°F.

Cut the potatoes into large sticks. Toss the sticks with the oil, then sprinkle them with salt and toss them again to coat them evenly. Place the potato sticks in a single layer in a nonstick pan. Bake for 20 minutes; turn them with a metal spatula, and bake them on the other side for an additional 20 minutes.

Nutritional Analysis

Per Serving

Calories (kcal)	115.9	Cholesterol (mg)	0.0
Total Fat (g)	3.6	Dietary Fiber (g)	2.4
Saturated Fat (g)	0.3	% Calories from Fat	27.9
Monounsaturated Fat (g)	2.0	Vitamin C (mg)	19.0
Polyunsaturated Fat (g)	1.1	Vitamin A (i.u.)	16,395.0

SWEET POTATO PANCAKES

*These pancakes are delicious by themselves but may be topped
with applesauce or nonfat yogurt and scallions. Like all sweet potato
dishes they are high in beta-carotene, and the cakes contain vitamin C
as well from the white potatoes.*

Makes 6 servings

1 cup grated white potatoes
(peeling optional)

1 cup grated sweet potatoes
(peeling optional)

½ teaspoon salt plus additional
for seasoning the potatoes

3 eggs, beaten

1 cup grated carrot

⅓ cup flour

¼ cup chopped fresh parsley

2 tablespoons finely chopped
yellow onion

1 tablespoon fresh lemon juice

Place the grated white and sweet potatoes in a colander, salt them lightly, and
let them drain for 15 minutes. Rinse the potatoes and squeeze out all the
liquid. Combine the potatoes with the remaining ingredients and mix well.

Heat a nonstick pan (or griddle lightly coated with cooking spray). Use
2 tablespoons batter for each pancake, frying the cakes over medium heat until
they're golden brown and crisp on both sides.

Serve the hot pancakes immediately.

Nutritional Analysis

Per Serving

Calories (kcal)	106.5	Cholesterol (mg)	92.0
Total Fat (g)	2.3	Dietary Fiber (g)	1.8
Saturated Fat (g)	0.7	% Calories from Fat	19.6
Monounsaturated Fat (g)	0.8	Vitamin C (mg)	16.0
Polyunsaturated Fat (g)	0.4	Vitamin A (i.u.)	7,981.0

SWEET POTATOES WITH APPLES

This is a lovely dish for holiday meals. The apples add a great contrast in texture, and the orange juice and peel blend the flavors together without making an overly sweet dish . . . and it gives you almost 200 percent of the RDA of vitamin A (beta-carotene).

Makes 8 servings

4 large sweet potatoes, unpeeled and quartered

½ cup brown sugar

¼ cup fresh orange juice

2 teaspoons grated orange peel

½ teaspoon ground cinnamon

2 large Granny Smith apples, unpeeled and sliced

2 tablespoons chilled butter

Preheat the oven to 350°F.

Gently boil the sweet potatoes in water for about 20 minutes, or until they're just tender. Drain the potatoes, allow them to cool slightly, then slice them into ½-inch-thick pieces.

Combine the brown sugar, orange juice, orange peel, and cinnamon. In a casserole dish, layer one-third of the potato slices, then one-third of the apple slices, and sprinkle the apples with one-third of the brown sugar mixture. Repeat to make three layers. Cut the butter into several pieces and distribute them on top of the sugar. Bake the casserole for 30 minutes, or until the potatoes and apples are tender.

Nutritional Analysis

Per Serving

Calories (kcal)	145.8	Cholesterol (mg)	8.0
Total Fat (g)	3.0	Dietary Fiber (g)	2.2
Saturated Fat (g)	1.8	% Calories from Fat	18.2
Monounsaturated Fat (g)	0.8	Vitamin C (mg)	17.0
Polyunsaturated Fat (g)	0.2	Vitamin A (i.u.)	9,501.0

Walnut-Stuffed Sweet Potatoes

This recipe is another holiday favorite, and it is especially wonderful with poultry or pork. It can be prepared a day ahead, offering a delicious and elegant dish with no last-minute work. The fact that it contains 378 percent of the RDA of vitamin A (beta-carotene) is a bonus.

Makes 4 servings

4 medium sweet potatoes,
  unpeeled

1 tablespoon butter

¼ cup fresh orange juice

½ teaspoon salt

¼ cup chopped walnuts

Preheat the oven to 375°F.

Bake the potatoes for 45 minutes to 1 hour, until they're fork-tender. Remove the potatoes but leave the oven on. Cut a long slice off the top of each potato and scoop out the center, leaving a shell thick enough to support the potato.

Mash the centers with a fork, then add the butter, orange juice, and salt, and mix the ingredients just to combine them. The mixture should be light and fluffy. Spoon the potato mixture back into the shells. Sprinkle the walnuts on top and bake the stuffed potatoes for 20 minutes or until they're heated through.

Nutritional Analysis

Per Serving

Calories (kcal)	141.7	Cholesterol (mg)	8.0
Total Fat (g)	4.2	Dietary Fiber (g)	2.9
Saturated Fat (g)	1.9	% Calories from Fat	26.1
Monounsaturated Fat (g)	1.1	Vitamin C (mg)	29.0
Polyunsaturated Fat (g)	0.9	Vitamin A (i.u.)	18,895.0

Pasta

CHILLED CHINESE NOODLES WITH SESAME OIL AND ORANGE

This recipe could also be served as a hot noodle dish. Simply heat the dressing ingredients and pour the mixture over the hot, drained noodles.

Makes 8 servings

12 ounces vermicelli

1 cup grated carrot

3 tablespoons low-sodium soy sauce

3 tablespoons sliced scallion

1 tablespoon rice wine vinegar

1 tablespoon fresh orange juice

1 tablespoon sesame oil (Asian variety)

½ tablespoon hot chili oil

1 teaspoon orange zest

1 teaspoon sugar

Cook the vermicelli according to the package directions until the pasta is tender, about 10 minutes. Drain the vermicelli very well and place it in a large bowl. Combine the remaining ingredients and toss the mixture with the "noodles." Chill the mixture. Toss it again just before serving.

Nutritional Analysis

Per Serving

Calories (kcal)	187.1	Cholesterol (mg)	0.0
Total Fat (g)	2.8	Dietary Fiber (g)	0.5
Saturated Fat (g)	0.3	% Calories from Fat	13.2
Monounsaturated Fat (g)	1.2	Vitamin C (mg)	4.0
Polyunsaturated Fat (g)	0.9	Vitamin A (i.u.)	3,451.0

Lasagna Pinwheels with Two Sauces

Don't be alarmed by the length of the ingredients list—everything is quickly combined. These pinwheels are well worth making. The two sauces add to the beautiful presentation of this dish.

Makes 10 servings

1 pound extra-wide lasagna noodles

2 cups low-fat (1%) cottage cheese

2 cups part-skim ricotta cheese

1 20-ounce package frozen spinach, defrosted and squeezed dry

1 teaspoon dried oregano

½ teaspoon chopped fresh basil

¾ teaspoon salt

¼ teaspoon black pepper

¼ teaspoon ground nutmeg

4 cups marinara sauce*

¼ cup low-fat (1%) milk

¼ cup nonfat yogurt

¼ teaspoon white pepper

Preheat the oven to 350°F.

Boil the lasagna for 10 minutes in a large pot. Drain the lasagna very carefully and pat it dry.

To make the filling, combine the cottage cheese, 1 cup of the ricotta, the spinach, oregano, basil, ½ teaspoon of the salt, the black pepper, and the nutmeg. Spread the filling along the length of each lasagna noodle and roll the noodles up.

Place 2 cups of the marinara sauce on the bottom of a 9" × 13" pan. Place the rolled noodles in the pan on their *ends* (with one "curly" end up) and spoon the remaining 2 cups marinara sauce over the top. Bake the lasagna rolls for 45 minutes. If they begin to brown, lay a piece of foil loosely over them.

---

*Use commercial sauce or Red Bell Pepper and Tomato Sauce from Chapter 8.

Combine the remaining 1 cup ricotta, the milk, yogurt, the remaining ¼ teaspoon salt, and the white pepper to make the white sauce.

Slice the cooked, rolled-up lasagna noodles. They will look like pinwheels.

Dish up the pinwheels, spooning some of the marinara over each, then top each with a spoonful of the white sauce.

Nutritional Analysis

Per Serving

Calories (kcal)	370.3	Cholesterol (mg)	20.0
Total Fat (g)	9.6	Dietary Fiber (g)	2.8
Saturated Fat (g)	3.9	% Calories from Fat	22.7
Monounsaturated Fat (g)	3.3	Vitamin C (mg)	27.0
Polyunsaturated Fat (g)	1.4	Vitamin A (i.u.)	5,639.0

LINGUINE WITH CLAM SAUCE

*This recipe has only 18.3 percent calories from fat
and a good amount of beta-carotene.*

Makes 8 servings

8 ounces linguine

3 7½-ounce cans clams

5 teaspoons olive oil

2 tablespoons butter

1 cup chopped carrot

½ cup finely chopped scallion

2 large cloves garlic, minced

1 cup clam juice

1 cup low-fat (1%) milk

½ cup finely chopped fresh
  parsley

¼ teaspoon pepper

Cook the linguine according to the package directions and drain it. While the pasta is cooking, prepare the clam sauce.

Drain the clams and reserve the juice. Heat the oil and butter in a large skillet, add the carrot and sauté the carrot for 5 minutes. Add the scallion and garlic and cook for 5 minutes more (don't let them brown). Add the reserved juice from the canned clams, the cup of bottled juice, and the milk. Boil the sauce for 10 minutes.

Just before serving, add the clams, parsley, and pepper to the sauce. Bring the sauce to a boil again and pour it over the hot linguine. Serve immediately.

Nutritional Analysis

Per Serving

Calories (kcal)	411.8	Cholesterol (mg)	49.0
Total Fat (g)	8.2	Dietary Fiber (g)	5.7
Saturated Fat (g)	2.6	% Calories from Fat	18.3
Monounsaturated Fat (g)	3.2	Vitamin C (mg)	24.0
Polyunsaturated Fat (g)	1.1	Vitamin A (i.u.)	4,236.0

Linguine with Watercress and Garlic

This is one of our easiest recipes and also one of our favorites. Everything works so well together, and the basic flavors of the ingredients come through beautifully. Also, these are ingredients that are usually easy to assemble at the last minute—you can substitute spinach if watercress is not available.

Makes 6 servings

1 pound linguine

3 tablespoons olive oil

2 cloves garlic, minced

2 cups washed and chopped watercress

½ teaspoon salt

¼ teaspoon pepper

¼ cup grated Parmesan or Asiago cheese

Cook the linguine according to the package directions. Drain the pasta and immediately toss it with the oil, garlic, watercress, salt, and pepper. Add the cheese and toss the ingredients gently. The linguine may be served immediately as a hot pasta dish but also works well as a chilled pasta salad (great if there are leftovers).

Nutritional Analysis

Per Serving

Calories (kcal)	362.0	Cholesterol (mg)	3.0
Total Fat (g)	9.2	Dietary Fiber (g)	2.1
Saturated Fat (g)	1.9	% Calories from Fat	23.1
Monounsaturated Fat (g)	5.5	Vitamin C (mg)	5.0
Polyunsaturated Fat (g)	1.1	Vitamin A (i.u.)	519.0

Noodle Pudding with Spinach and Sun-Dried Tomatoes

This pudding is as good in flavor as it is rich in vitamins.

Makes 6 servings

10 ounces whole wheat noodles

3 cups low-fat cottage cheese

½ cup chopped fresh parsley

¼ cup chopped sun-dried tomatoes

2 scallions, sliced

½ teaspoon salt

¼ teaspoon pepper

1 teaspoon paprika

1 teaspoon dried oregano

1 tablespoon olive oil

1½ cups plus 2 tablespoons vegetable broth

1 cup chopped yellow onion

2 cloves garlic, minced

3 tablespoons flour

1 10-ounce package chopped spinach, defrosted and drained

4 ounces grated mozzarella cheese, part skim

Preheat the oven to 350°F. Coat a 9" × 13" baking dish with cooking spray.

Cook the noodles according to the package directions until tender. Drain the noodles and spread them in the baking dish. Mix the cottage cheese, parsley, sun-dried tomatoes, scallions, salt, pepper, paprika, and oregano. Spread the cottage cheese mixture over the noodles.

Heat a large skillet to medium-high and melt the oil in the pan with the 2 tablespoons broth. Add the onion and garlic, reduce the heat to medium, and sauté the vegetables for 5 minutes. Add the flour and cook until the ingredients are blended, stirring constantly. Add the remaining 1½ cups broth and bring the mixture to a boil; reduce the heat and simmer for 5 minutes, stirring constantly. Add the spinach and stir to combine. Spoon the mixture over the noodles and cheese. Top it off with mozzarella and bake the pudding for 20 to 25 minutes. Serve the noodle pudding hot.

Nutritional Analysis

Per Serving

Calories (kcal)	444.7	Cholesterol (mg)	16.0
Total Fat (g)	11.1	Dietary Fiber (g)	6.9
Saturated Fat (g)	3.4	% Calories from Fat	21.8
Monounsaturated Fat (g)	3.3	Vitamin C (mg)	44.0
Polyunsaturated Fat (g)	1.0	Vitamin A (i.u.)	5,677.0

Sauces, Salad Dressings, and Condiments

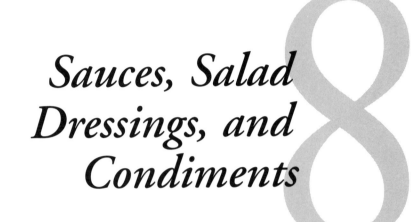

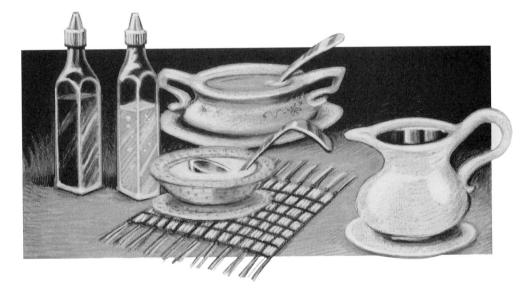

This is probably the most important chapter in the book. Nobody can live on skinless chicken and steamed vegetables 365 days a year.

If you are conscientious about following a reduced-fat diet, using only the leanest of meats and fish and removing the skin and fat from poultry, the results will certainly be healthful, but they also might leave you wanting something more. Plain meat, skinless chicken, bare poached fish, or simple vegetable dishes can all be complemented with additional flavor—herbs and spices. But you needn't stop there. A well-executed sauce offers limitless possibilities for interesting and satisfying entrees and will also dissipate the feeling that "something" is missing (that "something" being fat).

All of the sauces here are less than 30 percent calories from fat. Accomplishing this level was quite an undertaking, since most sauces and salad dressings (except for the fat-free bottled varieties) are usually 80 percent to 90 percent calories from fat.

The sauces in this chapter are designed to replace the fat with flavor, moisture, and general sensory appeal. The food looks as appetizing as it tastes delicious. The right sauce will dress up even the plainest piece of white fish, the loneliest slice of turkey breast, or the sparest slice of lean meat. (See the "Cooking Methods" sections in Chapter 4 for the best ways to prepare lean meats, fish, and poultry to ensure tenderness—even the most savory sauce cannot mask a leathery piece of meat or an overcooked piece of chicken or fish.)

This chapter features three categories of sauces: vegetable sauces, creamy-type sauces (lower in fat than typical cream sauce recipes), and herb-condiment sauces. Some of them contain small amounts of oil or butter, but the amounts are only a small fraction of the fat found in conventional sauces or the marbling of fatty meats.

You will notice that we have included a number of Asian-style dressings and sauces, since there are a wealth of Asian condiments that are very flavorful and also either low in fat or nonfat.

Because the dressings or sauces contain less than 30 percent calories from fat, you can use them generously. Remember, though, that they are not calorie free. If you are on a calorie-restricted diet, be sure to adhere to portion sizes.

Our version of a great marinara sauce (spaghetti sauce) is Red Bell Pepper and Tomato Sauce. Make a double batch and freeze the extra for quick pasta dinners.

To complement the taste of vegetables such as cauliflower, broccoli, carrots, or spinach, serve them with Spicy Ginger-Herb Dressing or Creamy Chive Sauce. These sauces contain less fat per tablespoon than butter or margarine.

Use some of the heartier sauces such as Madeira Sauce or Chicken Gravy to enhance turkey or chicken breasts. Mexican Green Chili Sauce or Sun-Dried Tomato Aioli can also perk up the plainest of foods, adding a zesty, spicy flavor.

Most of the sauces (except those containing yogurt, cheese, or mayonnaise) can be made ahead and frozen in small containers for fast dinners or meals for one. It takes only minutes to poach a piece of chicken, steam a fresh vegetable, and defrost one of the sauces to serve over both.

This chapter perhaps more than any other in the book demonstrates what interesting, varied, and delicious foods are available on a cancer risk-reduction diet. They will not leave you with deprivation.

Sauces

Chicken Gravy

The secret of this low-fat yet yummy gravy is the roasting of the flour.

Makes 6 servings

3 tablespoons flour
¼ cup low-fat (1%) milk
1 cup low-fat chicken broth

2 tablespoons finely chopped onion
¼ teaspoon white pepper

Set a heavy skillet over medium-high heat. Add the flour and cook, stirring constantly, for 5 to 10 minutes, until it turns a rich golden brown. (If the flour begins to smoke, reduce the heat to medium for a minute, then turn it back up.)

Combine the remaining ingredients in a saucepan and bring the mixture to a boil; add the flour all at once, incorporating it with a whisk. As soon as the gravy comes to a boil again, reduce the heat and simmer for 3 minutes.

Nutritional Analysis

Per Serving

Calories (kcal)	23.0	Cholesterol (mg)	0.0
Total Fat (g)	0.2	Dietary Fiber (g)	4.1
Saturated Fat (g)	0.1	% Calories from Fat	4.8
Monounsaturated Fat (g)	0.0	Vitamin C (mg)	0.0
Polyunsaturated Fat (g)	0.0	Vitamin A (i.u.)	21.0

CHILI SAUCE

Use this sauce on Mexican food such as chiles rellenos, burritos, and tacos, or to add interest without much fat to broiled or barbecued meat or chicken. It also adds interest to plain steamed vegetables.

Makes 6 servings (about 1⅓ cups)

1 8-ounce can tomato sauce

2 tablespoons canned, diced chilies

2 tablespoons red wine vinegar

1½ tablespoons finely chopped yellow onion

½ teaspoon ground cumin

Combine all the ingredients in a saucepan and simmer the contents for 15 minutes. Serve hot.

Nutritional Analysis

Per Serving

Calories (kcal)	15.4	Cholesterol (mg)	0.0
Total Fat (g)	0.1	Dietary Fiber (g)	0.6
Saturated Fat (g)	0.0	% Calories from Fat	6.9
Monounsaturated Fat (g)	0.0	Vitamin C (mg)	8.0
Polyunsaturated Fat (g)	0.0	Vitamin A (i.u.)	393.0

Cranberry-Tangerine Sauce

This cranberry sauce fills the house with a festive "holiday" aroma. Leftover, it is wonderful with cold turkey but is also fabulous with lean pork.

Makes 12 servings (4 cups)

2 tangerines, unpeeled and chopped coarse

2 cups water

1 12-ounce package cranberries

2 Granny Smith apples, unpeeled and chopped

1½ cups sugar

1 cup slivered almonds

Combine the tangerine and water in a large pan and cook the mixture rapidly until the peel is tender, about 20 minutes. Add the cranberries, apple, and sugar and bring the mixture to a boil over medium-low heat, stirring occasionally until the sugar is dissolved. Increase the heat and boil the sauce gently for 15 minutes. As the mixture thickens, stir it often to prevent sticking. Add the almonds and cook for 5 minutes longer.

This sauce may be made several days ahead, cooled, then covered and refrigerated. Remove it from the refrigerator in time to bring it to room temperature before serving.

Nutritional Analysis

Per Serving

Calories (kcal)	180.9	Cholesterol (mg)	0.0
Total Fat (g)	5.1	Dietary Fiber (g)	2.4
Saturated Fat (g)	0.5	% Calories from Fat	24.1
Monounsaturated Fat (g)	3.3	Vitamin C (mg)	8.0
Polyunsaturated Fat (g)	1.1	Vitamin A (i.u.)	105.0

CREAMY CHIVE SAUCE

This sauce is wonderful with fish and poultry. It is a very good match for vegetables and baked potatoes as well.

Makes 6 servings

½ cup nonfat yogurt

¼ cup part-skim ricotta cheese

1 tablespoon chopped fresh chives

¼ teaspoon salt

¼ teaspoon white pepper

⅛ teaspoon sugar

Process all the ingredients in a blender or food processor until the mixture is smooth.

Nutritional Analysis

Per Serving

Calories (kcal)	25.5	Cholesterol (mg)	3.0
Total Fat (g)	0.8	Dietary Fiber (g)	0.0
Saturated Fat (g)	0.5	% Calories from Fat	29.7
Monounsaturated Fat (g)	0.2	Vitamin C (mg)	0.0
Polyunsaturated Fat (g)	0.0	Vitamin A (i.u.)	67.0

Ginger Sauce

This sauce complements poultry of any kind or pork.
It also makes an interesting dip for chicken or nitrite-free turkey
sausages that have been grilled and sliced.

Makes 10 servings

1 16-ounce can apricot halves
   in juice, drained

⅓ cup corn syrup

¼ cup cider vinegar

¼ cup sliced scallion

½ teaspoon ground ginger

⅛ teaspoon cayenne

⅛ teaspoon allspice

Remove any pits from the apricots and place the apricots in a food processor or blender. Add the remaining ingredients and process the mixture until it's smooth. Place the mixture in a heavy saucepan and bring it to a boil; reduce the heat and simmer gently for 45 minutes.

Serve the sauce hot or at room temperature.

Nutritional Analysis

Per Serving

Calories (kcal)	45.2	Cholesterol (mg)	0.0
Total Fat (g)	0.1	Dietary Fiber (g)	0.7
Saturated Fat (g)	0.0	% Calories from Fat	1.4
Monounsaturated Fat (g)	0.0	Vitamin C (mg)	3.0
Polyunsaturated Fat (g)	0.0	Vitamin A (i.u.)	606.0

Greek Yogurt-Dill Sauce

One of our favorite meals is fresh salmon with this creamy sauce.
We serve a cucumber salad alongside or grate fresh peeled and seeded
cucumbers into the sauce for a coarser texture.

Makes 6 servings

1 cup nonfat yogurt

¼ cup sliced scallion

2 teaspoons fresh dill weed,
   or 1 teaspoon dried

½ teaspoon salt

¼ teaspoon white pepper

Combine all the ingredients. Serve the sauce with seafood, poultry, and vegetables and on salads.

Nutritional Analysis

Per Serving

Calories (kcal)	22.7	Cholesterol (mg)	1.0
Total Fat (g)	0.1	Dietary Fiber (g)	0.1
Saturated Fat (g)	0.0	% Calories from Fat	2.8
Monounsaturated Fat (g)	0.0	Vitamin C (mg)	2.0
Polyunsaturated Fat (g)	0.0	Vitamin A (i.u.)	21.0

MADEIRA SAUCE

This sauce can be made a couple of days ahead and refrigerated.
It works well with any plain entree.

Makes 16 servings (about 1 quart)

1 tablespoon butter

3 cups plus 3 tablespoons
low-fat chicken broth

¼ cup finely chopped yellow
onion

¾ cup Madeira

2 tablespoons cornstarch

¼ cup water

Heat a large skillet to medium and melt the butter and the 3 tablespoons chicken broth together. Add the onion and sauté for 5 minutes. Add the remaining 3 cups broth and the Madeira and bring the mixture to a boil. Stir and boil the mixture for 10 minutes. Mix the cornstarch and water and add the paste to the boiling sauce. Reduce the heat a bit and gently boil the sauce until it's thickened, about 5 minutes.

Nutritional Analysis

Per Serving

Calories (kcal)	26.1	Cholesterol (mg)	2.0
Total Fat (g)	0.7	Dietary Fiber (g)	0.1
Saturated Fat (g)	0.4	% Calories from Fat	29.0
Monounsaturated Fat (g)	0.2	Vitamin C (mg)	0.0
Polyunsaturated Fat (g)	0.0	Vitamin A (i.u.)	27.0

Mexican Green Chili Sauce

Use this sauce to pour over plain chicken or meat, or in Mexican food such as chiles rellenos, burritos, or enchiladas. It also makes a refreshing addition to vegetables or rice.

Makes 10 servings (about 4½ cups)

1 12-ounce can diced chilies

1½ cups low-fat chicken broth

10 large romaine lettuce leaves

1 teaspoon sugar

½ teaspoon ground cumin

½ teaspoon ground coriander

2 teaspoons olive oil

Combine all the ingredients, except the oil, in a food processor or blender and puree the mixture. Heat the oil in a large skillet and add the puree. Simmer the sauce for 5 minutes, or until it's thickened, stirring often.

Serve the green chili sauce hot or at room temperature.

Nutritional Analysis

Per Serving

Calories (kcal)	24.6	Cholesterol (mg)	0.0
Total Fat (g)	1.0	Dietary Fiber (g)	0.6
Saturated Fat (g)	0.1	% Calories from Fat	28.4
Monounsaturated Fat (g)	0.7	Vitamin C (mg)	63.0
Polyunsaturated Fat (g)	0.1	Vitamin A (i.u.)	455.0

Red Bell Pepper and Tomato Sauce

We call this our basic marinara sauce. Serve this versatile sauce on pasta, vegetables, poultry, or meat. It also makes a simple and delicious hors d'oeuvre when spooned on toasted French bread and topped with chopped fresh basil, shrimp, fresh tomato, Mediterranean olives, or anchovies.

Makes 8 servings (about 1¾ cups)

1 8-ounce can tomato sauce

1 7-ounce jar bell peppers, drained

1 scallion, minced

1 clove garlic, minced

1 tablespoon balsamic vinegar

2 teaspoons chopped fresh basil

1½ teaspoons olive oil

¼ teaspoon salt

Puree all the ingredients in a food processor or blender until the mixture is smooth. Serve the sauce at room temperature or gently heated.

Nutritional Analysis

Per Serving

Calories (kcal)	26.5	Cholesterol (mg)	0.0
Total Fat (g)	1.0	Dietary Fiber (g)	1.2
Saturated Fat (g)	0.1	% Calories from Fat	28.5
Monounsaturated Fat (g)	0.6	Vitamin C (mg)	25.0
Polyunsaturated Fat (g)	0.1	Vitamin A (i.u.)	491.0

Sun-Dried Tomato Aioli

In this aioli, a bit of mayonnaise is used, but the substance of the sauce comes from the potato, which blends the flavors of the garlic, sun-dried tomato, and basil rather than relying on a cupful of mayonnaise to do so. The texture is slightly different from that of traditional aioli. Use this on fish or poultry, as a dip for new vegetables, as a sauce for hot vegetables, or as a sandwich spread with tomatoes, cucumber, and red onion.

Makes 8 servings (about 1½ cups)

1 8-ounce baking potato
⅓ cup low-fat (1%) milk
2 teaspoons mayonnaise
3 large cloves garlic, minced
1½ tablespoons minced oil-free, sun-dried tomatoes*

1½ tablespoons minced fresh basil
1 teaspoon fresh lemon juice
¼ teaspoon sugar
¼ teaspoon salt
⅛ teaspoon white pepper

Peel the potato, cut it into cubes, and boil it until it's tender. Drain the potato and mash it with a fork until smooth (you should have about 1 cup). Add the milk to the potato and mix well. Add the remaining ingredients and stir to combine.

Allow the mixture to set at least 1 hour before serving. The aioli may be served at room temperature or gently heated.

_____

*As sun-dried tomatoes (not in oil) can be a bit "leathery," using scissors is a good way to cut them.

Nutritional Analysis

Per Serving

Calories (kcal)	34.8	Cholesterol (mg)	1.0
Total Fat (g)	1.2	Dietary Fiber (g)	0.4
Saturated Fat (g)	0.2	% Calories from Fat	28.9
Monounsaturated Fat (g)	0.3	Vitamin C (mg)	5.0
Polyunsaturated Fat (g)	0.5	Vitamin A (i.u.)	52.0

Salad Dressings

Asian Raspberry Vinegar Dressing

This dressing is rather light. It will coat your salad satisfactorily and add a wonderful flavor. To keep the content under 30 percent calories from fat, very little oil is used. However, you will not be disappointed with the intense flavor.

Makes 6 servings

1 teaspoon dry mustard

2 teaspoons water

¼ cup low-sodium chicken broth

1 teaspoon sugar

3 tablespoons raspberry vinegar (see Index)

2 tablespoons low-sodium soy sauce

½ teaspoon sesame oil (Asian variety)

Mix the dry mustard and water to form a paste; add the remaining ingredients and blend to combine.

Nutritional Analysis

Per Serving

Calories (kcal)	15.9	Cholesterol (mg)	0.0
Total Fat (g)	0.5	Dietary Fiber (g)	0.1
Saturated Fat (g)	0.1	% Calories from Fat	25.5
Monounsaturated Fat (g)	0.2	Vitamin C (mg)	0.0
Polyunsaturated Fat (g)	0.2	Vitamin A (i.u.)	0.0

CUCUMBER DRESSING

This is a refreshing dressing for chilled poached salmon or poultry.

Makes 8 servings (about 1⅓ cups)

1 medium cucumber	2 teaspoons red wine vinegar
1 clove garlic, minced	½ teaspoon salt
½ cup low-fat yogurt	¼ teaspoon sugar
1 tablespoon chopped scallion	⅛ teaspoon white pepper

Peel the cucumber and cut it in half lengthwise. Scoop out the seeds and grate the flesh. Squeeze out the excess liquid. Combine the remaining ingredients with the cucumber.

Store the dressing in the refrigerator.

Nutritional Analysis

Per Serving

Calories (kcal)	20.0	Cholesterol (mg)	1.0
Total Fat (g)	0.3	Dietary Fiber (g)	0.6
Saturated Fat (g)	0.2	% Calories from Fat	13.0
Monounsaturated Fat (g)	0.1	Vitamin C (mg)	4.0
Polyunsaturated Fat (g)	0.0	Vitamin A (i.u.)	169.0

Fruit Salad Dressing

*This is an excellent dressing for a fruit salad or drizzled on a platter
of fresh sliced fruits as a refreshing dessert.*

Makes 6 servings (about 1 cup)

¾ cup low-fat yogurt

¼ cup fresh orange juice

1 tablespoon honey

½ teaspoon dried mint flakes

Mix all the ingredients in a food processor or blender until smooth. Store the
dressing in the refrigerator.

Nutritional Analysis

Per Serving

Calories (kcal)	33.5	Cholesterol (mg)	2.0
Total Fat (g)	0.5	Dietary Fiber (g)	0.0
Saturated Fat (g)	0.3	% Calories from Fat	11.8
Monounsaturated Fat (g)	0.1	Vitamin C (mg)	5.0
Polyunsaturated Fat (g)	0.0	Vitamin A (i.u.)	37.0

GINGER-SOY DRESSING

You can also use this salad dressing with rice, pasta, vegetables (instead of butter), and baked potatoes (instead of sour cream).

Makes 4 servings

¼ cup rice wine vinegar

2 tablespoons low-sodium soy sauce

½ teaspoon water

⅜ teaspoon sesame oil (Asian variety)

¼ teaspoon finely minced fresh ginger

¼ teaspoon sugar

Whisk all the ingredients together vigorously in a large mixing bowl.

Nutritional Analysis

Per Serving

Calories (kcal)	11.7	Cholesterol (mg)	0.0
Total Fat (g)	0.4	Dietary Fiber (g)	0.11
Saturated Fat (g)	0.1	% Calories from Fat	29.4
Monounsaturated Fat (g)	0.2	Vitamin C (mg)	0.0
Polyunsaturated Fat (g)	0.0	Vitamin A (i.u.)	0.0

Hoisin-Orange Vinaigrette

*This vinaigrette has an unbelievably rich taste even though
the fat content is under 30 percent calories from fat.*

Makes 6 servings

¼ cup fresh orange juice

¼ cup low-sodium chicken
   broth

½ teaspoon finely chopped
   fresh ginger

1 tablespoon hoisin sauce

½ teaspoon dry mustard

2 teaspoons low-sodium
   soy sauce

Process all the ingredients in a blender or food processor until smooth.
Refrigerate the dressing for several hours or overnight.

Nutritional Analysis

Per Serving

Calories (kcal)	12.9	Cholesterol (mg)	0.0
Total Fat (g)	0.4	Dietary Fiber (g)	0.0
Saturated Fat (g)	0.1	% Calories from Fat	26.4
Monounsaturated Fat (g)	0.2	Vitamin C (mg)	6.0
Polyunsaturated Fat (g)	0.1	Vitamin A (i.u.)	3.0

MISO DRESSING

This is a perfect dressing to keep around for salads, vegetables, poultry, fish, rice, or even pasta. It's as delicious as it is versatile and very simple to make.

Makes 8 servings

½ cup water

⅓ cup miso

3 tablespoons low-sodium soy sauce

2 tablespoons rice wine vinegar

1 teaspoon brown sugar

Combine all the ingredients in a food processor or blender.

Nutritional Analysis

Per Serving

Calories (kcal)	29.9	Cholesterol (mg)	0.0
Total Fat (g)	0.7	Dietary Fiber (g)	0.5
Saturated Fat (g)	0.1	% Calories from Fat	20.4
Monounsaturated Fat (g)	0.2	Vitamin C (mg)	0.0
Polyunsaturated Fat (g)	0.4	Vitamin A (i.u.)	10.0

Raspberry Vinegar

*Raspberry vinegar may be used alone on salads or vegetables—it has such
a good flavor that oil is not missed. Make some for your own use,
and give the rest as hostess gifts in attractive bottles.*

Makes about 6 cups

1 pound raspberries, fresh or
frozen (without sugar)

¼ cup sugar

4 cups white wine vinegar

Combine all the ingredients in a nonreactive (nonmetallic) heavy saucepan.
Simmer the mixture gently for 10 minutes. Place the mixture in a large jar and
store it covered for 3 weeks.

Strain the mixture through a mesh strainer, pressing on the berries to extract
as much juice as possible. Strain it again through a coffee filter to get a bright,
clear vinegar. Transfer the liquid to attractive, clean bottles and store them
tightly covered.

Nutritional Analysis

Per Serving

Calories (kcal)	22.5	Cholesterol (mg)	0.0
Total Fat (g)	0.1	Dietary Fiber (g)	0.8
Saturated Fat (g)	0.0	% Calories from Fat	2.9
Monounsaturated Fat (g)	0.0	Vitamin C (mg)	5.0
Polyunsaturated Fat (g)	0.1	Vitamin A (i.u.)	2.0

Sour Cream–Style Dressing

*Use this dressing on baked potatoes or as a sauce for vegetables;
it works almost anywhere sour cream would—you can even try
a small spoonful on top of Mexican food.*

Makes 6 servings

⅔ cup low-fat yogurt

⅓ cup low-fat (1%) cottage
cheese

1 teaspoon fresh lemon juice

½ teaspoon salt

¼ teaspoon white pepper

Process all the ingredients in a food processor or blender until the mixture is
very smooth. Store the dressing in the refrigerator.

Nutritional Analysis

Per Serving

Calories (kcal)	25.5	Cholesterol (mg)	2.0
Total Fat (g)	0.5	Dietary Fiber (g)	0.0
Saturated Fat (g)	0.3	% Calories from Fat	18.3
Monounsaturated Fat (g)	0.1	Vitamin C (mg)	1.0
Polyunsaturated Fat (g)	0.0	Vitamin A (i.u.)	21.0

Spicy Ginger-Herb Dressing

Use this refreshing and spicy dressing on baked potatoes, seafood, poultry, salad, and especially spinach! (Heat the dressing for a "hot spinach salad.")

Makes 10 servings

1 tablespoon chopped fresh mint

¼ cup chopped fresh cilantro

1 cup nonfat yogurt

⅓ cup rice wine vinegar

1 tablespoon sugar

2 tablespoons canned, diced chilies

2 teaspoons fresh minced ginger

½ teaspoon salt

Puree all the ingredients in a food processor or blender.

Nutritional Analysis

Per Serving

Calories (kcal)	19.5	Cholesterol (mg)	0.0
Total Fat (g)	0.0	Dietary Fiber (g)	0.0
Saturated Fat (g)	0.0	% Calories from Fat	1.8
Monounsaturated Fat (g)	0.0	Vitamin C (mg)	4.0
Polyunsaturated Fat (g)	0.0	Vitamin A (i.u.)	22.0

Yogurt-Chutney Dressing

*This dressing is especially tasty on spinach, fruit, and chicken salads.
Splurge and buy an exotic chutney.*

Makes 6 servings (about 1 cup)

1 cup low-fat yogurt

3 tablespoons chutney

½ teaspoon curry powder

1 teaspoon canola oil

Chop the chutney and combine it with the remaining ingredients in a food processor or blender, processing until smooth. Store the dressing in the refrigerator.

Nutritional Analysis

Per Serving

Calories (kcal)	50.8	Cholesterol (mg)	2.0
Total Fat (g)	1.4	Dietary Fiber (g)	0.3
Saturated Fat (g)	0.4	% Calories from Fat	24.5
Monounsaturated Fat (g)	0.6	Vitamin C (mg)	1.0
Polyunsaturated Fat (g)	0.2	Vitamin A (i.u.)	96.0

Yogurt-Herb Dressing

This salad dressing also makes a wonderful sauce for poultry, vegetables, or seafood. Try it as a dip for crab claws instead of mayonnaise.

Makes 6 servings

1 cup nonfat yogurt

2 tablespoons white wine vinegar

½ teaspoon dried oregano

½ teaspoon salt

¼ teaspoon dried thyme

¼ teaspoon dried basil

¼ teaspoon pepper

¼ teaspoon garlic powder

Combine all the ingredients and allow the flavors to blend for at least 1 hour before using. Store the dressing in the refrigerator.

Nutritional Analysis

Per Serving

Calories (kcal)	23.1	Cholesterol (mg)	1.0
Total Fat (g)	0.1	Dietary Fiber (g)	0.1
Saturated Fat (g)	0.0	% Calories from Fat	2.7
Monounsaturated Fat (g)	0.0	Vitamin C (mg)	0.0
Polyunsaturated Fat (g)	0.0	Vitamin A (i.u.)	19.0

CONDIMENTS

Chardonnay Applesauce
with Sweet Onion and Thyme

Because traditional applesauce is sometimes too sweet to enjoy with savory dishes, we decided to make an applesauce that is savory, to match the entree. The combination of sweet and tart apples is a perfect balance to accompany most any dish.

Makes 8 servings

6 Granny Smith apples

6 Golden Delicious apples

1 cup water

1 cup finely chopped yellow onion

¼ cup chardonnay

¼ cup sugar

2 tablespoons butter

½ tablespoon finely chopped fresh thyme leaves

¼ teaspoon salt

Peel and core the apples and slice them about ⅛-inch thick. Place the apple slices in a heavy saucepan with the remaining ingredients, tossing gently to combine them without breaking up the apples too much. Bring the mixture to a boil, reduce the heat, and simmer the sauce, stirring occasionally, for 30 minutes, until most of the liquid is absorbed and the apples are soft but retain some shape.

Allow the applesauce to set before serving. (The mixture will thicken as it cools.)

Nutritional Analysis

Per Serving

Calories (kcal)	144.1	Cholesterol (mg)	8.0
Total Fat (g)	3.1	Dietary Fiber (g)	3.9
Saturated Fat (g)	1.9	% Calories from Fat	19.1
Monounsaturated Fat (g)	0.9	Vitamin C (mg)	9.0
Polyunsaturated Fat (g)	0.3	Vitamin A (i.u.)	107.0

CRANBERRY SALSA

This is not a sauce for the traditional holiday supper, but rather a sweet-and-tart salsa. It's a perfect accompaniment to pork, veal, and lamb, as well as poultry—a much better choice for cold meat or poultry on a buffet table than mayonnaise or sour cream sauces. It only has 0.9 percent calories from fat per serving.

Makes 8 servings

16-ounce can whole-cranberry sauce

¼ cup minced yellow onion

¼ cup chopped fresh cilantro

1 teaspoon orange zest

1 teaspoon red wine vinegar

½ teaspoon salt

Combine all the ingredients and mix well. The salsa is best if it's made several hours before serving. It may be made several days ahead and refrigerated.

Serve at room temperature.

Nutritional Analysis

Per Serving

Calories (kcal)	87.7	Cholesterol (mg)	0.0
Total Fat (g)	0.1	Dietary Fiber (g)	0.7
Saturated Fat (g)	0.0	% Calories from Fat	0.9
Monounsaturated Fat (g)	0.0	Vitamin C (mg)	3.0
Polyunsaturated Fat (g)	0.0	Vitamin A (i.u.)	25.0

CUCUMBER-MINT RAITA

In addition to being a wonderful accompaniment to Indian food, this raita is good with poultry, seafood, baked potatoes, and vegetables.

Makes 8 servings (about 2 cups)

1 cucumber, peeled

1 cup nonfat yogurt

¼ cup chopped fresh parsley

2 tablespoons chopped fresh mint

1 tablespoon canned, diced chilies

1 teaspoon lemon zest

½ teaspoon salt

¼ teaspoon white pepper

Cut the cucumber in half lengthwise and remove the seeds. Grate the flesh, then drain it for 30 minutes. Combine the cucumber with the remaining ingredients.

Nutritional Analysis

Per Serving

Calories (kcal)	26.7	Cholesterol (mg)	1.0
Total Fat (g)	0.2	Dietary Fiber (g)	0.7
Saturated Fat (g)	0.0	% Calories from Fat	5.1
Monounsaturated Fat (g)	0.0	Vitamin C (mg)	9.0
Polyunsaturated Fat (g)	0.0	Vitamin A (i.u.)	263.0

LEMON-GINGER APPLESAUCE

You can use a combination of apples for more depth of flavor. Mixing tart apples (such as Granny Smith), sweet apples (such as Golden Delicious), and apples with some tang (such as McIntosh) gives a wonderful balance.

Makes 12 servings (about 2 quarts)

12 large apples

1 cup water

2 teaspoons lemon zest

½ cup sugar

2 teaspoons minced ginger

Peel and core the apples, then coarsely chop them. Place the apples in a large, heavy saucepan with the water and lemon zest. Bring the mixture to a boil, reduce the heat, and gently boil the apples for 30 minutes, stirring occasionally. Add the sugar and ginger and continue cooking for 10 more minutes.

The applesauce may be pureed after cooking; however, a slightly chunky applesauce seems more homemade and much more interesting in both flavor and texture.

Nutritional Analysis

Per Serving

Calories (kcal)	107.4	Cholesterol (mg)	0.0
Total Fat (g)	0.5	Dietary Fiber (g)	3.5
Saturated Fat (g)	0.1	% Calories from Fat	3.5
Monounsaturated Fat (g)	0.0	Vitamin C (mg)	8.0
Polyunsaturated Fat (g)	0.1	Vitamin A (i.u.)	67.0

Roasted Balsamic Onions

These onions make a great low-fat garnish for plain vegetables, grilled chicken, or turkey sausages. Also try them as a topping for pizza.

Makes 6 servings (about 2 cups)

1½ pounds Maui, Vidalia, or red onions, sliced thin

4 cloves garlic, minced

2 teaspoons dried oregano

5 teaspoons olive oil

1 tablespoon balsamic vinegar

½ teaspoon sugar

¼ teaspoon salt

¼ teaspoon pepper

Preheat the oven to 400°F.

Combine the onion, garlic, and oregano in a 9" × 13" pan. Toss the mixture with the oil to coat the onion, then toss it with vinegar. Sprinkle the onion mixture with the sugar, salt, and pepper and toss all the ingredients well once again. Bake for 40 minutes.

Nutritional Analysis

Per Serving

Calories (kcal)	62.6	Cholesterol (mg)	0.0
Total Fat (g)	1.7	Dietary Fiber (g)	2.2
Saturated Fat (g)	0.2	% Calories from Fat	23.4
Monounsaturated Fat (g)	1.1	Vitamin C (mg)	8.0
Polyunsaturated Fat (g)	0.2	Vitamin A (i.u.)	35.0

Sweet and Savory Bakery

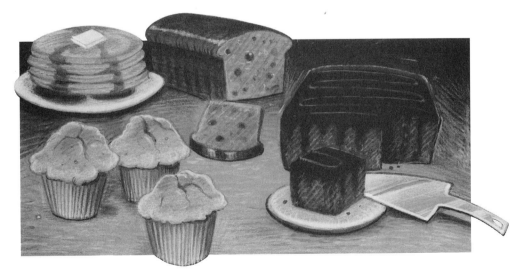

Sweet Bakery

Baking is an art separate from general cooking. Many people find that baking helps give them a feeling of well-being. The house is filled with fragrant scents, and "breaking bread" together fosters feelings of camaraderie.

Many of our selections from Sweet Bakery are great breakfast foods, especially if you have a sweet tooth. Some weekend brunch treats are Blueberry Pancakes, Norwegian Pancakes, Apple-Ginger Scones with Three-Citrus Zest, and Vanilla-Walnut Granola. Amor Polenta could be either a breakfast food or a dessert.

Cranberry-Orange-Zinfandel Bread is an example of a sweet yet tart bread. If you only have a few minutes for breakfast, give your children a slice of Oatmeal Breakfast Bread and a glass of low-fat (1%) milk or orange juice.

AMOR POLENTA

*This traditional Italian cake with its crispy exterior is a crowd pleaser.
The fresh strawberries are a wonderful presentation in color and texture
and contain a good amount of vitamin C. The fat has been
greatly reduced from the standard amor polenta.*

Makes 12 servings

4½ tablespoons butter,
   softened

1¼ cups sifted powdered sugar

1 teaspoon vanilla extract

1 egg, lightly beaten, plus
   2 lightly beaten egg whites

1¼ cups flour

⅓ cup polenta or cornmeal

1 teaspoon baking soda

3 cups sliced strawberries

Preheat the oven to 350°F. Lightly coat a loaf pan with cooking spray, and dust it with flour.

Cream the butter and sugar until the mixture has the texture of coarse crumbs (using a fork and your fingertips works best). Mix the vanilla with the egg and egg whites, add the liquids to the sugar mixture and whisk to combine.

Combine the flour, polenta, and baking soda and add the dry ingredients to the batter. Stir until all the ingredients are well combined. Transfer the batter to the loaf pan. Bake for 40 minutes. Let the polenta set for a few minutes on a rack, then turn it out of the pan.

May be served warm or at room temperature. Top each serving with ¼ cup of the strawberries.

Nutritional Analysis

Per Serving

Calories (kcal)	163.5	Cholesterol (mg)	28.0
Total Fat (g)	5.4	Dietary Fiber (g)	1.5
Saturated Fat (g)	3.1	% Calories from Fat	29.6
Monounsaturated Fat (g)	1.6	Vitamin C (mg)	20.0
Polyunsaturated Fat (g)	0.4	Vitamin A (i.u.)	226.0

Apple-Ginger Scones
with Three-Citrus Zest

*As tangerines are seasonal, lime zest may be substituted
if tangerines aren't available.*

Makes 8 servings

3 cups flour, plus additional
for dusting

7 tablespoons sugar

1 tablespoon baking powder

1½ teaspoons baking soda

¼ teaspoon salt

6 tablespoons cold butter, cut in
pieces

1 egg, slightly beaten

¾ cup plus 1 tablespoon low-fat
buttermilk

2 tablespoons minced fresh ginger

1½ teaspoons lemon zest

1½ teaspoons orange zest

1½ teaspoons tangerine zest
(or lime zest)

2 medium tart apples, unpeeled,
cored, and sliced

Preheat the oven to 425°F. Dust a baking sheet with flour.

Sift the 3 cups flour, 6 tablespoons of the sugar, the baking powder, baking
soda, and salt together into a large bowl or food processor. Cut the butter into
the dry ingredients with a fork or pastry blender or by using a food processor
until the mixture is the texture of coarse crumbs.

Mix the egg, the ¾ cup buttermilk, the ginger, and the citrus zest and add the
ingredients to the flour mixture. Stir or process just until a soft dough forms.
(Transfer the dough from the food processor to a bowl at this point.) Add the
apples and stir them into the dough, just until they're combined.

Transfer the dough to a floured board and pat it into a circle about 8 inches in
diameter. Brush the top with the remaining 1 tablespoon buttermilk and
sprinkle it with the remaining 1 tablespoon sugar. Cut the circle into eight
wedges and place them on the baking sheet. Bake the scones until they're
golden, about 20 minutes.

Nutritional Analysis

Per Serving

Calories (kcal)	326.4	Cholesterol (mg)	46.0
Total Fat (g)	9.9	Dietary Fiber (g)	2.3
Saturated Fat (g)	5.7	% Calories from Fat	27.0
Monounsaturated Fat (g)	2.8	Vitamin C (mg)	3.0
Polyunsaturated Fat (g)	0.6	Vitamin A (i.u.)	373.0

APRICOT BREAD

When they are in season, fresh apricots can be used for this bread. Be sure they are ripe, so that they have full flavor and will puree nicely.

Makes 12 servings

2 cups whole wheat flour, plus additional for dusting

½ cup brown sugar

2 teaspoons baking soda

1 teaspoon pumpkin pie spice or ground cinnamon

¼ teaspoon salt

1 32-ounce can apricot halves in juice, drained

2 eggs, slightly beaten

¼ cup canola oil

2 teaspoons vanilla extract

Preheat the oven to 350°F. Coat a loaf pan with cooking spray and dust with flour.

Mix the five dry ingredients together. Puree the apricots in a food processor or blender. Mix the apricot puree with the eggs, oil, and vanilla and add the liquid to the dry mixture, blending well (don't overmix).

Transfer the batter to the loaf pan and bake the bread for 55 minutes.

Set the pan on a rack for a few minutes, then remove the loaf from the pan and place it on the rack to cool.

Nutritional Analysis

Per Serving

Calories (kcal)	192.1	Cholesterol (mg)	31.0
Total Fat (g)	5.7	Dietary Fiber (g)	3.4
Saturated Fat (g)	0.6	% Calories from Fat	25.5
Monounsaturated Fat (g)	3.0	Vitamin C (mg)	4.0
Polyunsaturated Fat (g)	1.6	Vitamin A (i.u.)	1,324.0

BLACKBERRY MUFFINS

This batter may also be baked as one loaf, three miniloaves, or three dozen minimuffins. We find that people really like the minimuffins, as they can enjoy three muffins instead of just one. During the holidays, purchase disposable miniloaf pans and bake this as three loaves, then wrap them and tie them with a ribbon for gifts.

Makes 12 servings

2 cups flour

½ cup plus 2 tablespoons sugar

1 teaspoon baking powder

1 teaspoon baking soda

¼ teaspoon salt

8 ounces low-fat blueberry yogurt

⅓ cup fresh orange juice

2 tablespoons canola oil

1 teaspoon vanilla extract

1 egg plus 2 egg whites, slightly beaten

1 8-ounce package frozen unsweetened blackberries, defrosted

Preheat the oven to 400°F. Coat a 12-cup muffin tin with cooking spray.

Mix the flour, the ½ cup sugar, the baking powder, baking soda, and salt in a large bowl (if the berries are sweetened, use only ⅓ cup sugar). Combine the remaining ingredients, except the berries and the remaining 2 tablespoons sugar, and mix the liquid gently with the dry ingredients just until they're combined. Gently fold in the berries and their juice until they're barely blended with the batter. Spoon the batter into the muffin cups. Sprinkle the remaining 2 tablespoons sugar over the batter and bake the muffins for 15 minutes.

Nutritional Analysis

Per Serving

Calories (kcal)	179.6	Cholesterol (mg)	16.0
Total Fat (g)	3.1	Dietary Fiber (g)	1.6
Saturated Fat (g)	0.4	% Calories from Fat	15.7
Monounsaturated Fat (g)	1.6	Vitamin C (mg)	4.0
Polyunsaturated Fat (g)	0.9	Vitamin A (i.u.)	55.0

BLUEBERRY PANCAKES

These are buttery, as well as deliciously moist from the blueberries. Add a touch of pure maple syrup and you may have found your favorite pancakes. (They are also a good source of dietary fiber.)

Makes 6 servings

1 egg plus 2 egg whites

1¾ cups low-fat buttermilk

¼ cup lemon-flavored carbonated mineral water

¼ cup butter, melted and cooled

¾ cup all-purpose flour

¾ cup whole wheat flour

6 tablespoons sugar

2 teaspoons baking powder

1½ teaspoons baking soda

½ teaspoon salt

12 ounces blueberries

Beat the egg and egg whites with the buttermilk, mineral water, and butter until the liquids are well blended.

Combine the remaining ingredients, except the blueberries, and add the dry ingredients to the egg mixture, blending just to combine them. Fold in the blueberries.

Coat a griddle or skillet with cooking spray and heat it to medium-high. Spoon ¼ cup batter for each pancake onto the hot griddle. Cook the cakes for 3 minutes, then turn them over and cook the other side for 2 to 3 minutes more, until the pancakes are cooked through (add more cooking spray if needed). Cover cooked pancakes to keep them warm while cooking the rest.

Nutritional Analysis

Per Serving

Calories (kcal)	299.0	Cholesterol (mg)	53.0
Total Fat (g)	9.5	Dietary Fiber (g)	3.8
Saturated Fat (g)	5.6	% Calories from Fat	27.9
Monounsaturated Fat (g)	2.8	Vitamin C (mg)	8.0
Polyunsaturated Fat (g)	0.7	Vitamin A (i.u.)	386.0

Carrot-Zucchini Bread

This bread is moist and delicious. Serve it with low-fat cream cheese for a quick breakfast or snack.

Makes 12 servings

2 cups whole wheat flour	1 tablespoon vanilla extract
½ tablespoon ground cinnamon	2 eggs
2 teaspoons baking powder	½ cup low-fat (1%) milk
¼ teaspoon salt	1⅔ cups grated carrot
½ teaspoon ground allspice	1⅓ cups grated zucchini
⅔ cup brown sugar	1½ cups raisins
¼ cup canola oil	

Preheat the oven to 350°F. Coat a loaf pan with cooking spray.

Combine the six dry ingredients in a large mixing bowl. Mix the oil, vanilla, eggs, and milk in a blender or food processor until the liquids are combined.

Add the liquid to the dry ingredients and mix in the carrot, zucchini, and raisins until blended. Pour the batter into the loaf pan and bake the bread for 45 to 55 minutes, or until the top springs back when gently touched in the center.

Let the pan set for a few minutes, then remove the loaf and place it on a rack to cool.

Nutritional Analysis

Per Serving

Calories (kcal)	235.7	Cholesterol (mg)	31.0
Total Fat (g)	5.9	Dietary Fiber (g)	3.9
Saturated Fat (g)	0.7	% Calories from Fat	21.3
Monounsaturated Fat (g)	3.0	Vitamin C (mg)	3.0
Polyunsaturated Fat (g)	1.6	Vitamin A (i.u.)	3,937.0

CINNAMON-APPLE BREAD

Your family will love this bread served at a weekend brunch with apple butter.

Makes 12 servings

2 cups flour

⅓ cup brown sugar

1 teaspoon baking powder

1 teaspoon baking soda

1 teaspoon ground cinnamon

½ teaspoon ground nutmeg

¼ teaspoon salt

1 cup low-fat buttermilk

2 tablespoons vegetable oil

1 teaspoon vanilla extract

1 egg plus 2 egg whites, slightly beaten

2 medium apples, unpeeled and chopped

Preheat the oven to 350°F. Coat a loaf pan with cooking spray.

Mix the seven dry ingredients in a large bowl. Combine the remaining ingredients, except the apple, and gently mix the liquid with the dry ingredients just until they're combined. Gently fold in the apple. Transfer the batter to the pan. Bake the loaf for about 1 hour.

Set the pan on a rack for about 10 minutes, then remove the bread and place it on the rack to cool thoroughly. The loaf should come out of the pan in one piece. Do not allow the bread to "sweat" and become soggy by remaining in the pan.

Nutritional Analysis

Per Serving

Calories (kcal)	149.8	Cholesterol (mg)	16.0
Total Fat (g)	3.1	Dietary Fiber (g)	1.3
Saturated Fat (g)	0.5	% Calories from Fat	18.9
Monounsaturated Fat (g)	1.6	Vitamin C (mg)	1.0
Polyunsaturated Fat (g)	0.6	Vitamin A (i.u.)	34.0

CRANBERRY-ORANGE-ZINFANDEL BREAD

The beauty of this bread is that it is not as sweet as most other "quick breads,"
making it appealing to those who are not fond of sweet food in the morning.
It is also suitable as an appetizer with light cream cheese
or as a fall dessert with some apples and pears.

Makes 12 servings

2 tablespoons canola oil

1 egg, slightly beaten

2 cups flour

¾ cup sugar

2 teaspoons baking powder

½ teaspoon salt

½ teaspoon baking soda

½ cup chopped walnuts

1½ cups cranberries

⅓ cup fresh orange juice

¼ cup white zinfandel

Preheat the oven to 350°F. Coat a loaf pan with cooking spray.

In a large bowl, mix the oil and egg. Combine the flour, sugar, 1½ teaspoons of the baking powder, the salt, and baking soda. Mix the dry ingredients with the liquid, stirring just until they're combined (the mixture will be crumbly).

Fold in the walnuts and cranberries and gently combine them. Add the juice and zinfandel and stir until the ingredients are just blended. Pour the batter into the loaf pan and bake the bread for 1 hour, or until the top springs back when gently touched in the center.

Nutritional Analysis

Per Serving

Calories (kcal)	170.3	Cholesterol (mg)	15.0
Total Fat (g)	3.6	Dietary Fiber (g)	1.2
Saturated Fat (g)	0.3	% Calories from Fat	19.1
Monounsaturated Fat (g)	1.7	Vitamin C (mg)	5.0
Polyunsaturated Fat (g)	1.3	Vitamin A (i.u.)	34.0

DRIED CRANBERRY BREAD

For a light bread, mix the moist and dry ingredients together very gently just until they're combined. The bread will be heavy if you overmix.

Makes 12 servings

2 cups flour

⅔ cup brown sugar

¼ cup cornmeal

1 tablespoon baking powder

1 teaspoon baking soda

¼ teaspoon salt

8 ounces low-fat vanilla yogurt

¼ cup low-fat (1%) milk

2 tablespoons butter, melted and cooled

1 teaspoon vanilla extract

1 egg plus 2 egg whites, slightly beaten

1 cup dried cranberries

Preheat the oven to 350°F. Coat a loaf pan with cooking spray.

Mix the six dry ingredients in a large bowl. Combine the remaining ingredients, except the cranberries, and gently mix the liquid with the dry ingredients just until they're combined. Gently fold in the cranberries just until blended. Transfer the batter to the loaf pan and bake the bread for about 1 hour.

Nutritional Analysis

Per Serving

Calories (kcal)	185.7	Cholesterol (mg)	21.0
Total Fat (g)	2.8	Dietary Fiber (g)	1.5
Saturated Fat (g)	1.5	% Calories from Fat	13.7
Monounsaturated Fat (g)	0.8	Vitamin C (mg)	3.0
Polyunsaturated Fat (g)	0.3	Vitamin A (i.u.)	134.0

Norwegian Pancakes

These pancakes are delicious, foolproof, and easy to make. They have only 10 percent calories from fat, good fiber, and vitamin C.

Makes 6 servings

3 cups low-fat buttermilk	1 tablespoon sugar
1 egg, slightly beaten	2 teaspoons baking soda
1 cup all-purpose flour	⅛ teaspoon salt
1 cup whole wheat flour	3 cups sliced strawberries

Whisk together the buttermilk and egg in a large bowl. Combine the flours, sugar, baking soda, and salt and add the dry ingredients to the liquid mixture, stirring to combine them.

Coat a griddle or skillet with cooking spray and heat it to medium-high. Spoon ¼ cup batter for each pancake onto the hot griddle. Cook the cakes for 3 minutes, then turn them over and cook the other side for 2 to 3 minutes more, until the pancakes are cooked through (add more cooking spray if needed).

Serve the pancakes with the fresh strawberries. Add a small amount of syrup if desired.

Nutritional Analysis

Per Serving

Calories (kcal)	231.3	Cholesterol (mg)	35.0
Total Fat (g)	2.6	Dietary Fiber (g)	4.7
Saturated Fat (g)	0.9	% Calories from Fat	10.0
Monounsaturated Fat (g)	0.7	Vitamin C (mg)	41.0
Polyunsaturated Fat (g)	0.5	Vitamin A (i.u.)	64.0

Oatmeal Breakfast Bread

This is a wonderful breakfast even for picky children.
Serve a slice with a glass of low-fat (1%) milk and sliced strawberries.

Makes 12 servings

4 tablespoons butter, at room
   temperature

1 cup rolled oats

1¼ cups fresh orange juice

2 eggs, beaten

1 banana, mashed

1½ cups dried cranberries

⅔ cup all-purpose flour

⅔ cup whole wheat flour

⅓ cup granulated sugar

⅓ cup brown sugar

1 teaspoon baking soda

1 teaspoon ground cinnamon

½ teaspoon ground allspice

¼ teaspoon salt

Place the butter and oats in a large bowl. Heat the orange juice almost to boiling and pour the juice over the butter and oats. Allow the contents to set for 20 minutes.

Preheat the oven to 350°F.

Coat a 9" × 13" pan with cooking spray. Add the remaining ingredients to the bowl and mix thoroughly. Pour the batter into the pan and bake the bread for 35 minutes.

Serve hot right from the pan.

Nutritional Analysis

Per Serving

Calories (kcal)	193.1	Cholesterol (mg)	41.0
Total Fat (g)	5.3	Dietary Fiber (g)	3.2
Saturated Fat (g)	2.7	% Calories from Fat	23.8
Monounsaturated Fat (g)	1.5	Vitamin C (mg)	17.0
Polyunsaturated Fat (g)	0.5	Vitamin A (i.u.)	218.0

Raspberry-Lemon Muffins

These muffins, as well as most of the sweet breads and muffins in this chapter, have only a moderate amount of sugar. We like the flavor of the berries or other fruit to come through rather than being masked by excessive amounts of sugar.

Makes 12 servings

2 cups flour

½ cup brown sugar

1 tablespoon baking powder

1 teaspoon baking soda

¼ teaspoon salt

8 ounces low-fat raspberry yogurt

2 tablespoons butter, melted and cooled

1 tablespoon lemon zest

1 teaspoon vanilla extract

1 egg plus 2 egg whites, slightly beaten

1 12-ounce package frozen raspberries, defrosted but not drained

Preheat the oven to 400°F. Coat a 12-cup muffin tin with cooking spray.

Mix the five dry ingredients in a large bowl (if the berries are sweetened, use only ⅓ cup brown sugar). Combine the yogurt, butter, lemon zest, vanilla, and egg and egg whites and gently mix the liquid with the dry ingredients, just until they're combined. Gently fold in the berries and their juice, until the fruit is barely blended with the batter.

Spoon the batter into the muffin cups. Bake the muffins for 15 minutes, or until the tops spring back when lightly touched in the center.

Nutritional Analysis

Per Serving

Calories (kcal)	184.4	Cholesterol (mg)	21.0
Total Fat (g)	2.7	Dietary Fiber (g)	1.9
Saturated Fat (g)	1.5	% Calories from Fat	13.2
Monounsaturated Fat (g)	0.8	Vitamin C (mg)	5.0
Polyunsaturated Fat (g)	0.2	Vitamin A (i.u.)	120.0

STRAWBERRY BREAD

This bread is a wonderful use for fresh strawberries in season. The amount of oil has been reduced to keep this usually high-fat bread within the bounds of good nutrition. Just one slice has 25 percent of the RDA of vitamin C!

Makes 24 servings (2 loaves)

24 ounces strawberries

2 eggs plus 4 egg whites

7 tablespoons canola oil

1 teaspoon vanilla extract

3¼ cups flour

2 cups sugar

1 tablespoon ground cinnamon

1 teaspoon baking soda

¾ teaspoon salt

Preheat the oven to 350°F. Coat two loaf pans with cooking spray and dust them with flour.

Finely chop the berries. In a large bowl, beat the eggs and egg whites, then stir in the oil, vanilla, and berries.

Combine the remaining ingredients and add them to the berry mixture, stirring just to combine (don't overmix). Divide the batter evenly between the pans. Bake the loaves for 1½ hours.

Set the pans on a wire rack for a few minutes, then remove the loaves and place them on the rack to cool.

Nutritional Analysis

Per Serving

Calories (kcal)	178.6	Cholesterol (mg)	15.0
Total Fat (g)	4.6	Dietary Fiber (g)	1.2
Saturated Fat (g)	0.4	% Calories from Fat	22.9
Monounsaturated Fat (g)	2.5	Vitamin C (mg)	15.0
Polyunsaturated Fat (g)	1.3	Vitamin A (i.u.)	30.0

VANILLA-WALNUT GRANOLA

A granola without oil or butter? Absolutely! Even though no oil is used in this delicious granola, it is rich with flavor from the vanilla, pure maple syrup, and walnuts. This is a fun one to experiment with . . . for Vanilla-Orange-Walnut Granola use 1 teaspoon each vanilla and orange extracts; or add some dried cranberries or blueberries; try a full tablespoon of vanilla for an even richer flavor; use an equal amount of slivered almonds instead of the walnuts; or substitute honey for the maple syrup.

Makes 16 servings (about 8 cups)

6 cups rolled oats

2 cups chopped walnuts

½ cup 100% maple syrup

2 teaspoons vanilla extract

⅛ teaspoon salt

Preheat the oven to 325°F.

In a large bowl, combine the oats and walnuts. Heat the syrup, vanilla, and salt in a saucepan, or in the microwave for 90 seconds, until warm. Thoroughly mix the warm liquid with the oats and nuts. Spread the granola on two cookie sheets. Bake for 20 minutes, stirring after 10 minutes to prevent burning. The granola is done when it turns a light golden color.

Let the granola cool before serving.

Nutritional Analysis

Per Serving

Calories (kcal)	166.9	Cholesterol (mg)	0.0
Total Fat (g)	4.0	Dietary Fiber (g)	3.4
Saturated Fat (g)	0.5	% Calories from Fat	21.4
Monounsaturated Fat (g)	1.1	Vitamin C (mg)	0.0
Polyunsaturated Fat (g)	2.1	Vitamin A (i.u.)	42.0

Walnut-Coffee Bread

This is another wonderful breakfast treat. Serve it with fresh fruit.

Makes 12 servings

1¾ cups flour

⅓ cup brown sugar

½ cup granulated sugar

2 tablespoons instant espresso
coffee powder

½ teaspoon salt

1 egg plus 2 egg whites,
slightly beaten

¾ cup low-fat (1%) milk

2 tablespoons butter, melted
and cooled

1 teaspoon vanilla extract

3 tablespoons chopped
walnuts

Preheat the oven to 350°F. Coat a loaf pan with cooking spray.

Mix the flour, brown sugar, ¼ cup of the granulated sugar, the coffee powder, and salt in a large bowl. Combine the egg and egg whites, milk, butter, and vanilla and gently mix the liquid with the dry ingredients, just until they're combined.

Pour the batter into the loaf pan and sprinkle it with the remaining ¼ cup sugar and the walnuts. Bake the loaf for about 1 hour.

The bread is done if the top springs back when gently touched in the center, or when a toothpick inserted in the center comes out clean. You may need to adjust the cooking time a little, depending on your oven.

Nutritional Analysis

Per Serving

Calories (kcal)	159.5	Cholesterol (mg)	21.0
Total Fat (g)	2.9	Dietary Fiber (g)	0.5
Saturated Fat (g)	1.4	% Calories from Fat	16.1
Monounsaturated Fat (g)	0.8	Vitamin C (mg)	0.0
Polyunsaturated Fat (g)	0.4	Vitamin A (i.u.)	126.0

Savory Bakery

In our Savory Bakery we have taken eight classic recipes, lowered the fat, and punched up the flavor with herbs and spices. (See Chapter 2 for recommendations of great bread and soup combinations.) French Bread–Pecan Stuffing is a flavorful variation of holiday poultry stuffing. It can be baked alone if you like your "dressing" crunchy or put it into the turkey for a moister texture.

This section offers delicious recipes with low-fat content compared with regular breads, muffins, and scones. Their taste is incomparable. However, we do suggest these foods as *occasional* treats, especially if you are trying to lose weight. Most people just don't need extra carbohydrates at meals every day. Also, don't assume that the lower fat content means you can gobble a second or third helping. Adhere to suggested portion sizes.

BRAN MUFFINS

*The addition of low-fat yogurt and crushed pineapple
gives these high-fiber muffins wonderful texture and taste.*

Makes 24 servings

2 cups whole wheat flour	1 cup low-fat yogurt
1 cup 100% bran cereal	½ cup low-fat (1%) milk
¼ cup wheat germ	1 egg, slightly beaten
1½ tablespoons baking powder	¼ cup honey
1½ teaspoons baking soda	2 tablespoons canola oil
½ teaspoon salt	1 8-ounce can crushed
1½ tablespoons ground cinnamon	pineapple in juice
½ cup brown sugar	3 cups raisins

Preheat the oven to 400°F. Coat two 12-cup muffin tins with cooking spray.

Combine the first eight ingredients (flour through brown sugar). Mix the remaining ingredients and add the liquid to the dry ingredients. Mix until the batter is blended.

Divide the mixture among the 24 muffin cups. Bake the muffins for 25 minutes.

Allow the muffins to cool in the tins for a few minutes, then remove them and place them on a rack.

Nutritional Analysis

Per Serving

Calories (kcal)	155.8	Cholesterol (mg)	8.0
Total Fat (g)	2.1	Dietary Fiber (g)	3.2
Saturated Fat (g)	0.3	% Calories from Fat	10.9
Monounsaturated Fat (g)	0.5	Vitamin C (mg)	4.0
Polyunsaturated Fat (g)	1.3	Vitamin A (i.u.)	34.0

CORN BREAD

This recipe could also be baked as corn muffins. Transfer the batter to 12 muffin cups that have been coated with cooking spray and bake the tin for 15 minutes, or until the tops spring back when gently touched in the center. Serve the bread or muffins with one of our hearty soups from Chapter 2.

Makes 12 servings

1 cup cornmeal	½ teaspoon salt
1 cup flour	1 egg, slightly beaten
3 tablespoons sugar	1 cup low-fat (1%) milk
1 tablespoon baking powder	3 tablespoons canola oil

Preheat the oven to 400°F. Coat a loaf pan with cooking spray.

Combine the cornmeal, flour, sugar, baking powder, and salt in a large bowl. Beat the egg, milk, and oil together and add the liquid mixture to the dry ingredients. Mix just until all the ingredients are combined. Pour the batter into the loaf pan and bake the bread for 35 minutes.

Let the bread cool slightly before cutting.

Nutritional Analysis

Per Serving

Calories (kcal)	136.6	Cholesterol (mg)	16.0
Total Fat (g)	4.3	Dietary Fiber (g)	1.1
Saturated Fat (g)	0.5	% Calories from Fat	28.2
Monounsaturated Fat (g)	2.3	Vitamin C (mg)	0.0
Polyunsaturated Fat (g)	1.2	Vitamin A (i.u.)	112.0

French Bread–Pecan Stuffing

This stuffing may be made a day ahead, cooled completely, covered, and refrigerated. If it is part of a holiday meal, it may be placed in the oven alongside the turkey for the last hour. It may also be used to stuff a turkey or chicken. Or serve it as a side dish with lean pork or poultry. It is as delicious as it is easy to prepare.

Makes 12 servings

2 tablespoons butter

1 cup low-fat chicken broth

2 cups chopped yellow onion

2 cups chopped celery

1 pound French bread, cut into small cubes

1½ cups chopped fresh parsley

¼ cup chopped pecans

1 tablespoon poultry seasoning

½ teaspoon salt

½ teaspoon pepper

Preheat the oven to 350°F.

Heat the butter and broth in a large skillet over medium-high heat. Add the onion and celery and sauté the vegetables until they're softened, about 10 minutes. Remove the pan from the heat and add the remaining ingredients, tossing to combine them well. (More broth may be added if a moister stuffing is desired.) Transfer the mixture to a casserole dish and bake the stuffing for 1 hour.

Nutritional Analysis

Per Serving

Calories (kcal)	147.3	Cholesterol (mg)	5.0
Total Fat (g)	4.0	Dietary Fiber (g)	2.3
Saturated Fat (g)	1.5	% Calories from Fat	23.7
Monounsaturated Fat (g)	1.5	Vitamin C (mg)	13.0
Polyunsaturated Fat (g)	0.6	Vitamin A (i.u.)	500.0

Fresh Herb Muffins

Savory rather than sweet muffins are an unusual idea and a delightful change from ordinary dinner rolls or bread. These chive- and parsley-studded muffins are a nice complement to any meal, and they make a wonderful snack, or light lunch when paired with a salad. Try baking them in miniature muffin tins and serving them as an hors d'oeuvre.

Makes 12 servings

2 cups flour

2 teaspoons sugar

2 teaspoons baking powder

½ teaspoon salt

1 egg

1 cup low-fat (1%) milk

3 tablespoons butter, melted and cooled

⅓ cup chopped fresh chives

⅓ cup chopped fresh parsley

Preheat the oven to 400°F. Coat a 12-cup muffin tin with cooking spray.

Combine the flour, sugar, baking powder, and salt in a large bowl. Whisk together the egg, milk, butter, chives, and parsley and add the liquid mixture to the dry ingredients. Mix just until combined.

Pour the batter into the muffin cups and bake the muffins for 20 to 25 minutes, or until the tops spring back when gently touched in the center.

Nutritional Analysis

Per Serving

Calories (kcal)	118.8	Cholesterol (mg)	24.0
Total Fat (g)	3.6	Dietary Fiber (g)	0.7
Saturated Fat (g)	2.0	% Calories from Fat	27.8
Monounsaturated Fat (g)	1.0	Vitamin C (mg)	3.0
Polyunsaturated Fat (g)	0.2	Vitamin A (i.u.)	316.0

Garlic-Herb Bread

Although this bread isn't dripping with butter as is usually the case with garlic bread, it is delicious. There is enough butter to make it seem like the high-fat version, and the herbs and cheese give it lots of extra flavor and texture.

Makes 10 servings

1 loaf French bread

2½ tablespoons butter, at room temperature

4 cloves garlic, minced

5 tablespoons low-fat chicken broth

1 cup chopped fresh parsley

¼ teaspoon dried oregano

¼ teaspoon dried thyme

¼ teaspoon chopped fresh basil

½ cup grated Parmesan or Asiago cheese

Paprika

Preheat the oven to 400°F.

Split the bread lengthwise. Using a fork, combine the butter with the garlic until the mixture is fluffy. Add the broth, herbs, and cheese and blend thoroughly. Spread the mixture on the bread halves and sprinkle each half with paprika. Place the loaf on a baking sheet and bake for 10 minutes.

Nutritional Analysis

Per Serving

Calories (kcal)	176.9	Cholesterol (mg)	24.6
Total Fat (g)	5.8	Dietary Fiber (g)	1.5
Saturated Fat (g)	3.0	% Calories from Fat	29.3
Monounsaturated Fat (g)	1.8	Vitamin C (mg)	8.0
Polyunsaturated Fat (g)	0.4	Vitamin A (i.u.)	462.0

Irish Soda Bread

This is very simple bread to make—it involves no rising and only 2 to 4 minutes of kneading. Make this bread for Saint Patrick's Day (some plain, some with caraway seeds, and some with raisins) or enjoy it anytime.

Makes 16 servings (2 loaves)

4 cups flour, plus additional for dusting

½ cup sugar

1 teaspoon baking soda

1 teaspoon cream of tartar

¾ teaspoon salt

1¾ cups plus 2 teaspoons low-fat buttermilk

6 tablespoons butter, melted and cooled

Preheat the oven to 375°F. Coat a baking sheet with cooking spray and lightly flour it.

Combine the 4 cups flour, the sugar, baking soda, cream of tartar, and salt in a large bowl. Add the 1¾ cups buttermilk and the butter and mix well. Transfer the dough to a lightly floured surface (sprinkle the dough with additional flour if it's too sticky to handle). Knead for 2 minutes, or until the dough is firm.

Shape the dough into two round loaves. Rub each loaf with 1 teaspoon of the remaining buttermilk, then sprinkle each lightly with flour. Cut an X into the top of each loaf with a knife or scissors. Place the loaves on the baking sheet and bake the bread for 1 hour, or until the crust is a deep golden brown.

Variations

- For Caraway Bread, add 2 tablespoons caraway seeds along with the dry ingredients.
- For Raisin Bread, add 1 cup raisins along with the dry ingredients.

Nutritional Analysis

Per Serving

Calories (kcal)	186.8	Cholesterol (mg)	12.0
Total Fat (g)	4.8	Dietary Fiber (g)	0.9
Saturated Fat (g)	2.8	% Calories from Fat	23.3
Monounsaturated Fat (g)	1.3	Vitamin C (mg)	0.0
Polyunsaturated Fat (g)	0.3	Vitamin A (i.u.)	161.0

Mini Scallion-Cheese Scones

These are fabulous. They seem as if they must be loaded with fat, but they are not. You can bake these during the holidays and place them in an attractive basket to present as a hostess gift.

Makes 24 servings (24 scones)

1¼ cups flour, plus additional for dusting

½ teaspoon baking powder

⅛ teaspoon baking soda

⅛ teaspoon salt

2 teaspoons cold butter, cut in pieces

1 egg, beaten

⅓ cup nonfat yogurt

¼ cup minced scallion

¼ cup minced red onion

2 ounces grated sharp cheddar cheese

Preheat the oven to 400°F. Coat a baking sheet with cooking spray.

Combine the 1¼ cups flour, the baking powder, baking soda, and salt in a large bowl. Cut the butter into the dry ingredients until the pieces are the size of coarse crumbs. Add the egg and yogurt, mixing just until the ingredients are combined. Stir in the onion and cheese. The dough will be stiff, so use your hands to mix.

Turn the dough out onto a floured board and pat it into an 8-inch circle. Cut the circle into 24 triangles, which will be long and narrow. Place the triangles on the baking sheet and bake the scones for 15 minutes.

Nutritional Analysis

Per Serving

Calories (kcal)	41.3	Cholesterol (mg)	11.0
Total Fat (g)	1.3	Dietary Fiber (g)	0.2
Saturated Fat (g)	0.8	% Calories from Fat	29.6
Monounsaturated Fat (g)	0.4	Vitamin C (mg)	0.0
Polyunsaturated Fat (g)	0.01	Vitamin A (i.u.)	52.0

OAT BRAN MUFFINS

These high-fiber muffins are also high in taste and moisture from the addition of low-fat yogurt and crushed pineapple.

Makes 24 servings

2 cups whole wheat flour

1 cup oat bran

¼ cup wheat germ

1½ tablespoons baking powder

1½ teaspoons baking soda

½ teaspoon salt

1½ tablespoons cinnamon

½ cup brown sugar

1 cup nonfat yogurt

½ cup low-fat (1%) milk

1 egg, slightly beaten

¼ cup honey

2 tablespoons canola oil

1 8-ounce can crushed pineapple, undrained

3 cups raisins

Preheat the oven to 400°F. Coat two 12-cup muffin tins with cooking spray.

Combine the eight dry ingredients. Whisk together the yogurt, milk, egg, honey, oil, pineapple, and raisins and add the liquid mixture to the dry ingredients. Mix the batter just until all the ingredients are blended.

Divide the batter among the 24 muffin cups. Bake the muffins for 18 minutes, or until the tops spring back when gently touched in the center.

Allow the tins to set for a few minutes, then remove the muffins and place them on a rack to cool.

Nutritional Analysis

Per Serving

Calories (kcal)	157.5	Cholesterol (mg)	8.0
Total Fat (g)	2.1	Dietary Fiber (g)	2.9
Saturated Fat (g)	0.3	% Calories from Fat	10.6
Monounsaturated Fat (g)	0.9	Vitamin C (mg)	2.0
Polyunsaturated Fat (g)	0.6	Vitamin A (i.u.)	28.0

More Luscious Desserts

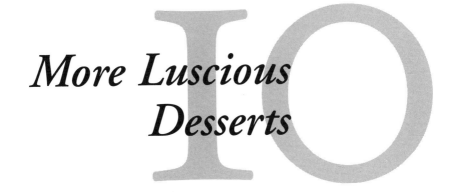

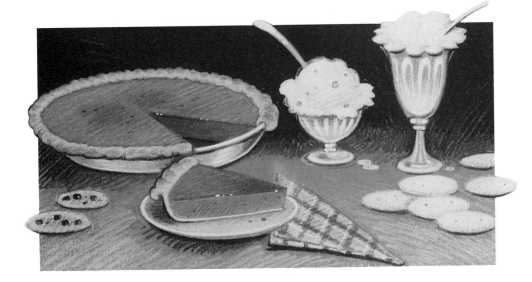

Dessert, the most whimsical and frivolous course of all, tempts the sweet tooth in all of us. Who can resist ending a meal with a luscious dessert? (Nobody we know, authors included!) This chapter is dedicated to those of you who immediately scan a restaurant menu for the dessert listings even before you have decided on an entree.

"Luscious" doesn't have to mean desserts *prohibitively* laden with fat or sugar. There are an abundance of recipes on a cancer risk-reduction eating plan that are also higher in vitamins and fiber and up to 60 percent lower in fat than usual dessert offerings.

We have not made any "foolers" in this chapter. There is no fake cheese-cake made with nonfat cottage cheese. We do have an ice-cream cake recipe that uses frozen yogurt. However, today frozen yogurt is as delicious as low-fat ice cream. We do use small amounts of butter, cream, and, of course, regular sugar. All of the desserts adhere to the requirement of no more than 30 percent calories from fat. However, some of the offerings contain a significant number of calories. Others have much lower caloric content.

Indeed, the dessert course should be viewed as a treat, and not a daily accompaniment to lunch or dinner. Pay attention to portion sizes, especially if you are trying to lose weight. We in no way suggest that these dishes can be eaten all the time. Eat dessert less often, unless it is a piece of fresh fruit. But when the occasion calls for a fabulous, satisfying dessert, you will not be disappointed with our selections.

Poached Winter Fruits with Blueberry Caviar makes an elegant fruit presentation. It has only 8.2 percent calories from fat and contains a good amount of vitamin C and dietary fiber. Double-Raspberry Chocolate "Tostadas" are also low in fat and contain 164 percent of the RDA of vitamin C and have a whopping 7.9 grams of dietary fiber (more than half the recommended daily amount suggested by the American Cancer Society).

If cake is your favorite, try Blackberry Coulis Cake with Grand Marnier Cream or Persimmon Cake with Orange-Ginger Cream. The latter has 17.7 percent calories from fat and almost 100 percent of the RDA of vitamin C.

For a holiday dessert, try Pumpkin Pie with Oatmeal Cookie Crust. This is a winner, especially with the children. For lunch-box treats, pack Cinnamon-Sugar Tortilla Chips or Sugar Cookies.

Egg whites contain no fat and are a good source of protein. They are the base ingredient for two elegant desserts, Hazelnut Meringue with Raspberry

Cream and Three-Citrus Meringue Tart. (The latter contains only 172.8 calories per serving.)

For a formal party, present your Viennese table using Chocolate Mousse, Lemon Bars, Six-Layer Torte with Lemon Curd and Strawberries (low in fat and high in vitamin C), and Apple Crisp.

We hope this rich variety of full-flavored desserts has convinced any lover of sweets that it is possible to have desserts that are good-tasting and that adhere to the guidelines of a cancer risk-reduction diet when eaten in moderation.

Ambrosia

This dessert deserves its name, boasting lovely flavor, color, and texture. It contains 10.3 percent calories from fat and 5.8 grams of fiber.

Makes 4 servings

2 tablespoons sesame seeds

½ cup low-fat yogurt

¼ cup honey

3 oranges, peeled

2 bananas, peeled

2 green apples, peeled

2 cups seedless grapes

Toast the sesame seeds by heating them in an ungreased frying pan for 5 minutes, shaking the pan frequently, until they're golden brown. Allow the seeds to cool.

Mix the yogurt and honey together to make the dressing.

Cut the oranges, bananas, and apples into bite-size cubes. Halve the grapes and gently toss all the fruit together right away to retain their color (the oranges will help prevent the other fruit from darkening).

Drizzle the dressing over the fruit and gently toss the mixture, taking care not to bruise the fruit. Sprinkle the sesame seeds on top.

Nutritional Analysis

Per Serving

Calories (kcal)	261.1	Cholesterol (mg)	2.0
Total Fat (g)	3.3	Dietary Fiber (g)	5.8
Saturated Fat (g)	0.8	% Calories from Fat	10.3
Monounsaturated Fat (g)	1.1	Vitamin C (mg)	51.0
Polyunsaturated Fat (g)	1.2	Vitamin A (i.u.)	376.0

APPLE-BRANDY COMPOTE

The elegance of this dessert belies the fact that it is low in fat and high in fiber.

Makes 8 servings

2 cups water

⅔ cup granulated sugar

1 teaspoon fresh lemon juice

3 pounds green apples,
   unpeeled and sliced

3 tablespoons brandy

1 teaspoon canola oil

¼ cup wheat germ

¼ teaspoon orange zest

½ cup plain low-fat yogurt

1 teaspoon ground cinnamon

½ teaspoon ground nutmeg

4 teaspoons brown sugar

Bring the water to a boil in a large pot; add the granulated sugar and lemon juice and return the pot to a boil. When the sugar has dissolved, add the apple slices, reduce the heat to medium, and simmer the mixture for about 20 minutes, gently stirring often to keep it from burning. (The apple slices will become almost transparent.) Stir in the brandy.

Mold

Using a pastry brush, brush a 4-cup mold or dish with the oil. Fit a piece of wax paper into the bottom of the mold, then turn the paper over so that both sides are coated with oil. Combine the wheat germ and orange zest and sprinkle the mixture over the wax paper on the bottom of the mold. Add the apple mixture. Chill the mold for several hours.

Yogurt Topping

Mix the yogurt with the cinnamon, nutmeg, and brown sugar. To unmold the compote, dip the mold briefly into hot water, run a knife around the edge, and reverse the compote onto a serving dish. Remove the wax paper. Slice the compote into eight portions, and top each with 1 tablespoon of the yogurt mixture.

Nutritional Analysis

Per Serving

Calories (kcal)	191.1	Cholesterol (mg)	1.0
Total Fat (g)	1.4	Dietary Fiber (g)	3.9
Saturated Fat (g)	0.4	% Calories from Fat	6.6
Monounsaturated Fat (g)	0.5	Vitamin C (mg)	7.0
Polyunsaturated Fat (g)	0.6	Vitamin A (i.u.)	11.0

APPLE-CRANBERRY COBBLER

This is one of our favorite desserts. Lemon zest adds interest to this apple-"infused" cobbler studded with piquant cranberries that burst in your mouth. Serve it warm.

Makes 10 servings

6 medium Granny Smith apples, unpeeled

1 cup cranberries

1¼ cups brown sugar

⅓ cup plus ¾ cup flour

1¼ teaspoons ground cinnamon

1 tablespoon lemon zest

¼ teaspoon salt

⅛ teaspoon ground nutmeg

5 tablespoons butter

Preheat the oven to 350°F. Coat a 9" × 13" pan with cooking spray.

Cobbler Filling

Remove the cores and coarsely chop the apples. Toss the apple with the cranberries, ½ cup of the brown sugar, the ⅓ cup flour, 1 teaspoon of the cinnamon, and the lemon zest. Place the mixture in the pan.

Cinnamon Topping

Mix the remaining ¾ cup each of flour and brown sugar, the salt, the remaining ¼ teaspoon cinnamon, and the nutmeg. Cut the butter into the flour mixture with a pastry blender or fork until the mixture is the texture of coarse crumbs.

Sprinkle the topping over the apple filling. Bake the cobbler for 30 minutes.

Nutritional Analysis

Per Serving

Calories (kcal)	246.1	Cholesterol (mg)	15.0
Total Fat (g)	5.9	Dietary Fiber (g)	2.6
Saturated Fat (g)	3.6	% Calories from Fat	21.0
Monounsaturated Fat (g)	1.7	Vitamin C (mg)	6.0
Polyunsaturated Fat (g)	0.4	Vitamin A (i.u.)	220.0

Apple Crisp

This is a fabulous fall dessert when crisp apples are at their best. It takes only minutes to make and may be enjoyed with a spoonful of low-fat fruit yogurt for extra appeal. (Try serving it warm topped with chilled raspberry or lemon yogurt.)

Makes 12 servings

9 medium green apples, unpeeled and sliced

3 tablespoons fresh lemon juice

1½ cups rolled oats

1 cup brown sugar

¾ cup flour

6 tablespoons butter, melted

1½ teaspoons ground cinnamon

Preheat the oven to 375°F.

Toss the apple slices with the lemon juice and place the mixture in a 9" × 13" pan. Combine the remaining ingredients and sprinkle the mixture evenly over the apple filling. Bake for 30 minutes.

Nutritional Analysis

Per Serving

Calories (kcal)	234.7	Cholesterol (mg)	15.0
Total Fat (g)	6.5	Dietary Fiber (g)	3.4
Saturated Fat (g)	3.7	% Calories from Fat	24.2
Monounsaturated Fat (g)	1.9	Vitamin C (mg)	6.0
Polyunsaturated Fat (g)	0.6	Vitamin A (i.u.)	225.0

Apple-Ginger Cake with Tangerine Cream

This low-fat dessert derives its texture and flavor from fruit.

Makes 10 servings

1 egg, slightly beaten
¼ cup canola oil
1 teaspoon fresh minced ginger
3 large apples, unpeeled and chopped coarse
1 cup flour
1 teaspoon baking soda
½ teaspoon plus ⅛ teaspoon salt
½ cup brown sugar

½ cup plus 2½ tablespoons granulated sugar
1½ teaspoons ground cinnamon
½ cup Grape-Nuts
2 teaspoons cornstarch
1½ tablespoons tangerine juice
¼ cup water
½ teaspoon tangerine zest
¼ cup whipping cream

Apple Cake

Preheat the oven to 350°F. Coat a 9" × 13" pan with cooking spray.

Mix the egg, oil, and ginger and toss the mixture with the apple. Combine the flour, baking soda, the ½ teaspoon salt, the brown sugar, the ½ cup granulated sugar, and the cinnamon and stir the dry ingredients into the apple mixture. Add the Grape-Nuts (the batter will be stiff). Spread the batter in the pan and bake the cake for 35 minutes, or until the top springs back when gently touched in the center.

Tangerine Cream

Combine the remaining 2½ tablespoons granulated sugar, the cornstarch, the remaining ⅛ teaspoon salt, the tangerine juice, water, and tangerine zest in a small saucepan. Cook the mixture over medium heat, stirring constantly, until the liquid is thick and clear. Gently boil the sauce for 1 minute. Remove the pan from the heat and let the contents cool. Whip the cream until it's stiff and fold it into the cooled tangerine mixture.

Serve the topping over the warm cake.

Nutritional Analysis

Per Serving

Calories (kcal)	269.5	Cholesterol (mg)	26.0
Total Fat (g)	8.9	Dietary Fiber (g)	2.6
Saturated Fat (g)	2.0	% Calories from Fat	29.0
Monounsaturated Fat (g)	4.2	Vitamin C (mg)	3.0
Polyunsaturated Fat (g)	2.0	Vitamin A (i.u.)	146.0

Blackberry Cantaloupe

*This simple dessert has jewel-like colors and boasts a wealth of vitamins
and fiber—and is very low in fat as a bonus.*

Makes 6 servings

1 pound blackberries, fresh or
frozen

¼ cup sugar

2 tablespoons cornstarch

2 tablespoons water

½ teaspoon vanilla extract

2 teaspoons fresh lemon juice

2 teaspoons blackberry liqueur
(or brandy)

1 large cantaloupe, peeled and
seeded

12 mint sprigs

Reserve 18 blackberries for the garnish, and heat the remaining berries and the
sugar to a boil in a heavy pan (if you're using frozen sweetened blackberries,
use only 2 tablespoons sugar). Mix the cornstarch with the water and vanilla
and add the paste to the boiling blackberry mixture.

Cook the sauce over medium heat, stirring constantly, for 10 minutes, or until it's
thickened. Let the sauce cool, then add the lemon juice and blackberry liqueur.

Pour the blackberry sauce into six individual dishes or one serving dish. Slice the
cantaloupe and place the sections on top of the sauce, overlapping them in an
attractive design. Garnish each serving with the mint sprigs and reserved berries.

Nutritional Analysis

Per Serving

Calories (kcal)	103.8	Cholesterol (mg)	44.0
Total Fat (g)	0.4	Dietary Fiber (g)	4.0
Saturated Fat (g)	0.0	% Calories from Fat	3.5
Monounsaturated Fat (g)	0.1	Vitamin C (mg)	136.0
Polyunsaturated Fat (g)	0.1	Vitamin A (i.u.)	1,583.0

BLACKBERRY COULIS CAKE
WITH GRAND MARNIER CREAM

Serve the blackberry coulis warm for a delightful temperature contrast.

Makes 10 servings

1 egg plus 1 egg white

1 cup low-fat (1%) milk

2½ cups flour

1¾ cups sugar

½ teaspoon salt

1 tablespoon baking powder

½ cup butter, melted and cooled

1 cup plain nonfat yogurt

2 tablespoons frozen lemonade concentrate

2 tablespoons Grand Marnier

1 tablespoon cornstarch

1 tablespoon water

1 pound blackberries, fresh or frozen

White Cake

Preheat the oven to 375°F. Coat a 9" × 13" pan with cooking spray.

Beat together the egg and egg white and the milk. In a separate bowl, combine the flour, 1½ cups of the sugar, the salt, baking powder, and butter. Combine both mixtures and blend well. Transfer the batter to the pan and bake the cake for 30 minutes.

Cream and Coulis

Meanwhile, whisk together the yogurt, lemonade concentrate, Grand Marnier, and 2 tablespoons of the remaining sugar. Cover the mixture and refrigerate it.

Mix the cornstarch with the water. In a saucepan combine the berries, the remaining 2 tablespoons sugar, and the cornstarch mixture. Bring the pot to a boil; immediately reduce the heat to low and simmer the sauce for 5 minutes. Keep the coulis warm until serving time.

To serve, ladle an equal amount of the hot blackberry coulis onto each plate. Top the coulis with a slice of cake, then garnish each serving with a spoonful of chilled Grand Marnier cream.

Nutritional Analysis

Per Serving

Calories (kcal)	403.2	Cholesterol (mg)	44.0
Total Fat (g)	10.3	Dietary Fiber (g)	3.2
Saturated Fat (g)	6.0	% Calories from Fat	23.0
Monounsaturated Fat (g)	2.9	Vitamin C (mg)	10.0
Polyunsaturated Fat (g)	0.6	Vitamin A (i.u.)	496.0

Chocolate Mousse

*For those who feel that it isn't dessert unless it's chocolate, try this mousse
topped with raspberry sauce and dotted with a spoonful of whipped cream.
The trick here, which you can try with some of your own recipes, is using
extra cocoa to enrich the flavor. (Use a top-quality chocolate.) Gelatin
compensates for the texture lost when most of the half-and-half
is replaced with whole milk and evaporated skim milk.*

*This is an excellent example of the principles of low-fat cooking; punch up
the flavor so that fat isn't missed, and compensate with other ingredients
(in this case, gelatin) for some of the change in texture.*

Makes 6 servings

9 tablespoons sugar	1⅓ cups whole milk
⅓ cup unsweetened cocoa	2 egg yolks
4 tablespoons cornstarch	1½ teaspoons vanilla extract
1½ teaspoons unflavored gelatin	10 ounces raspberries, fresh or frozen
⅓ cup half-and-half	2 tablespoons water
1 cup evaporated skim milk	1 tablespoon whipping cream

Mousse

Sift 6 tablespoons of the sugar, the cocoa, 2 tablespoons of the cornstarch, and
the gelatin into a heavy pan. Whisk in the half-and-half, evaporated skim
milk, and whole milk. Cook the mixture over medium heat for 10 minutes,
whisking constantly (reduce the heat if the mixture starts to simmer). Pour
about ½ cup of the hot mixture into a bowl, add the egg yolks, whisk the
mixture, then pour it back into the pan. Cook the contents over the lowest
heat setting, whisking constantly, for 4 minutes.

Remove the pan from the heat and whisk in the vanilla. Allow the mousse to
cool to room temperature, stirring occasionally to prevent a film from form-
ing. Divide the mousse into six 6-ounce serving dishes, cover each dish with
plastic wrap placed right on the surface of the mousse, and refrigerate the covered servings at least 2 hours or overnight.

Raspberry Sauce

Just before serving, make the sauce by bringing the raspberries and the remaining 3 tablespoons sugar to a boil in a saucepan. Blend the remaining 2 tablespoons cornstarch and water and add the mixture to the raspberries. Immediately reduce the heat to low and cook the syrup for 5 minutes. Remove the pan from the heat and keep the contents warm until serving time (or reheat later).

Whip the cream with a small wire whisk until it has some body (it doesn't have to be stiff). Remove the plastic wrap from the mousse, cover each portion with one-sixth of the warm sauce, then top it with a spoon of the whipped cream.

Nutritional Analysis

Per Serving

Calories (kcal)	240.8	Cholesterol (mg)	88.0
Total Fat (g)	6.8	Dietary Fiber (g)	2.1
Saturated Fat (g)	3.4	% Calories from Fat	24.2
Monounsaturated Fat (g)	2.0	Vitamin C (mg)	13.0
Polyunsaturated Fat (g)	0.5	Vitamin A (i.u.)	496.0

Chocolate Raspberry "Ice-Cream" Cake

Chocolate frozen yogurt tucked between layers of angel food cake, studded with fresh raspberries, and splashed with raspberry puree . . . a delight in color and flavor. All for only 17.2 percent fat calories, instead of the usual ice-cream cake with at least 46 percent calories from fat.

Makes 10 servings

1 12-ounce angel food cake

24 ounces low-fat chocolate frozen yogurt (3 cups)

12 ounces fresh raspberries

1 tablespoon sugar

1 tablespoon brandy

Slice the cake horizontally into three layers. Soften the frozen yogurt a bit, then spread one-third on the bottom layer of cake. Cover the yogurt with one-quarter of the raspberries. Repeat two more layers of cake, frozen yogurt, and raspberries.

In a food processor or blender, puree the remaining one-quarter of the raspberries with the sugar and brandy. Spoon the puree over the top of the cake, allowing sauce to drizzle down the side. Freeze the cake until it's firm, 30 to 60 minutes.

Cut the cake in slices to serve. (The cake can remain in the freezer for several hours, but if solidly frozen, it should set a few minutes at room temperature before serving time so the berries lose their frostiness.)

Nutritional Analysis

Per Serving

Calories (kcal)	220.5	Cholesterol (mg)	3.0
Total Fat (g)	4.4	Dietary Fiber (g)	1.5
Saturated Fat (g)	2.5	% Calories from Fat	17.2
Monounsaturated Fat (g)	1.2	Vitamin C (mg)	8.0
Polyunsaturated Fat (g)	0.3	Vitamin A (i.u.)	113.0

Cinnamon-Sugar Tortilla Chips

These are simple to make—a great dessert that you can serve with fresh fruit, and a sure favorite for a children's snack.

Makes 6 servings

6 8-inch flour tortillas

1½ teaspoons canola oil

2 tablespoons sugar

1 tablespoon ground cinnamon

¼ teaspoon ground nutmeg

Preheat the oven to 350°F.

Brush both sides of each tortilla with ¼ teaspoon oil. Combine the sugar, cinnamon, and nutmeg and sprinkle the mixture evenly over one side of each tortilla. Cut the tortillas into quarters and place the sections on a baking sheet. Bake the tortilla chips for 15 minutes.

Nutritional Analysis

Per Serving

Calories (kcal)	143.4	Cholesterol (mg)	0.0
Total Fat (g)	3.7	Dietary Fiber (g)	1.7
Saturated Fat (g)	0.5	% Calories from Fat	23.1
Monounsaturated Fat (g)	1.7	Vitamin C (mg)	0.0
Polyunsaturated Fat (g)	1.3	Vitamin A (i.u.)	3.0

CRANBERRY-GINGERSNAP "ICE-CREAM" PIE

The contrast in flavor, texture, and color makes this dessert so interesting. It is also simple to make. The bright red cranberry-orange topping covers a creamy, vanilla frozen yogurt filling that rests on a crispy, tasty gingersnap crust. Although we may think of cranberries for the holidays, this pie is a perfect summer dessert.

Makes 8 servings

½ cup crushed gingersnaps (about 10 cookies)

⅔ cup dry unseasoned bread crumbs

2 tablespoons butter, melted and cooled

1 tablespoon plus 2 teaspoons fresh orange juice

4 cups low-fat vanilla frozen yogurt

1 16-ounce can whole-cranberry sauce

1 tablespoon orange zest

1 teaspoon vanilla extract

Preheat the oven to 350°F.

Crush the gingersnaps in a food processor until they're the texture of coarse crumbs. Combine the gingersnap crumbs with the bread crumbs. Combine the butter with the 2 teaspoons orange juice, then add the liquid to the crumbs and mix thoroughly (fingertips work well here). Firmly press the gingersnap crust into a 10-inch pie pan and bake it for 10 minutes.

Allow the crust to cool, then fill it with the yogurt, smoothing the top. Freeze the pie until the yogurt is firm, about 4 hours.

Combine the cranberry sauce with the orange zest, the remaining 1 tablespoon orange juice, and the vanilla. Pour the mixture over the pie. Freeze the pie for a minimum of 5 hours.

This dessert is best if served the day it is made but may be frozen overnight (freeze until solid, about 4 hours, then cover it well with foil).

Nutritional Analysis

Per Serving

Calories (kcal)	327.3	Cholesterol (mg)	9.0
Total Fat (g)	8.8	Dietary Fiber (g)	1.4
Saturated Fat (g)	4.6	% Calories from Fat	27.7
Monounsaturated Fat (g)	3.1	Vitamin C (mg)	5.0
Polyunsaturated Fat (g)	0.6	Vitamin A (i.u.)	285.0

CRÈME CARAMEL WITH GRAND MARNIER

Even though it is simple to prepare, this is an elegant dessert. Using milk instead of cream brings the fat level down to the range of acceptable fat content. Using two egg whites and three eggs instead of six eggs also makes a difference in the amount of fat and cholesterol without compromising the quality of the custard.

Makes 4 servings

1 cup sugar

¼ cup water

1½ tablespoons orange zest

1 tablespoon Grand Marnier

2 cups milk

3 eggs plus 2 egg whites

1 teaspoon vanilla extract

To make the caramel sauce, place ½ cup of the sugar and 3 tablespoons of the water in a heavy saucepan. Boil the mixture over medium heat without stirring for 6 to 8 minutes, or until the sugar is golden brown. Combine the remaining 1 tablespoon water, the orange zest, and the Grand Marnier and add the mixture to the pan. Cook the sauce over medium heat for 5 minutes, stirring constantly. Pour the caramel sauce into the bottom of a 4-cup oven-proof dish or soufflé mold, tilting to evenly coat the base.

Preheat the oven to 350°F.

To make the custard, heat the milk in a heavy pan until bubbles form around the edge. Cover the pan to keep the milk hot. Beat the remaining ingredients together, then whisk the mixture into the hot milk. Pour the custard into the caramel-coated dish. Place the dish in a baking pan and fill the pan with enough hot water to reach halfway up the sides. Bake the custard for 30 minutes. Let the custard cool, then refrigerate it for 1 hour.

To serve, loosen the edges of the custard with a knife, cover the top with a deep plate, such as a pie dish, and turn the mold upside down—letting the caramel sauce flow over the custard.

Nutritional Analysis

Per Serving

Calories (kcal)	341.5	Cholesterol (mg)	154.0
Total Fat (g)	7.3	Dietary Fiber (g)	1.0
Saturated Fat (g)	3.5	% Calories from Fat	19.4
Monounsaturated Fat (g)	2.4	Vitamin C (mg)	4.0
Polyunsaturated Fat (g)	0.6	Vitamin A (i.u.)	366.0

Double-Raspberry Chocolate "Tostadas"

This is a fun dessert for the kids to help make as well as a delicious and unusual one. The chocolate tostadas make a great base for the raspberry frozen yogurt, and the raspberry sauce tops it all off with wonderful color and texture. And all this for only 13.5 percent calories from fat!

Makes 6 servings

1½ cups raspberries, fresh or frozen plus 18 additional for garnish

⅓ cup raspberry jam (top-quality)

1 tablespoon Tia Maria or other liqueur

¾ cup flour, plus additional for dusting

3 tablespoons unsweetened cocoa powder

¼ cup sugar

½ teaspoon baking powder

4 teaspoons vegetable shortening

4 tablespoons cold water

3 pints low-fat frozen raspberry yogurt

6 mint sprigs

To make the raspberry sauce, place the 1½ cups raspberries, the jam, and Tia Maria in a food processor or blender and process the ingredients until the mixture is smooth. Set the sauce aside.

In a food processor, mix the ¾ cup flour, cocoa, sugar, and baking powder until the ingredients are blended. Add the shortening and process the mixture on pulse (on and off) until the texture becomes sandy (as in making pie dough). Add the water and process just until the dough becomes a ball.

Knead the dough for 30 seconds on a lightly floured board. Cover the dough and set it aside for 30 minutes. Shape the dough into six rounds, cover it again, and set it aside for another 30 minutes.

Preheat the oven to 350°F. Coat a 6-cup muffin tin with cooking spray.

Roll the rounds of dough into 4-inch circles on a floured board. Place each circle over a muffin cup and fold the excess dough outward to make an edge. Bake the "tostadas" for 10 minutes.

Set each "tostada" on a serving plate and fill the shells with one-sixth of the yogurt. Drizzle the raspberry sauce over the top and garnish with the mint sprigs and the remaining raspberries.

Nutritional Analysis

Per Serving

Calories (kcal)	467.0	Cholesterol (mg)	8.0
Total Fat (g)	7.5	Dietary Fiber (g)	7.9
Saturated Fat (g)	2.7	% Calories from Fat	13.5
Monounsaturated Fat (g)	2.1	Vitamin C (mg)	98.0
Polyunsaturated Fat (g)	1.6	Vitamin A (i.u.)	584.0

FRESH PEACH SHORTCAKE

Whipped cream? On a healthful eating plan? Yes, when each portion contains only 2.4 teaspoons. This, of course, is an occasional treat.

You will see variations of this "lemon cream" used with several desserts in this book because it's a wonderful topping that carries other flavorings to enhance each particular dish. It is truly like whipped cream. The trick is that instead of using straight whipped cream, we use a small amount of freshly whipped cream that gets its body from the cornstarch-thickened syrup.

Makes 10 servings

1 egg plus 1 egg white

1 cup low-fat (1%) milk

½ cup butter, melted and cooled

2½ cups flour

1½ cups plus ⅔ cup sugar

¾ teaspoon salt

1 tablespoon baking powder

2 tablespoons cornstarch

⅓ cup fresh lemon juice

1 cup water

1 tablespoon lemon zest

2 pounds fresh peaches, unpeeled and chilled

½ cup whipping cream

Shortcake

Preheat the oven to 375°F. Coat a 9" × 13" pan with cooking spray.

Beat together the egg and egg white, milk, and butter. In a separate bowl, combine the flour, the 1½ cups sugar, ½ teaspoon of the salt, and the baking powder. Add the dry ingredients to the egg mixture and stir to combine.

Pour the batter into the pan and bake the cake for 30 minutes. Let the cake set in the pan for 5 minutes, then turn it out onto a rectangular tray. Let it cool for another 5 minutes, then slice it horizontally into two layers. Cool the layers completely on a rack.

Lemon Cream Sauce

While the cake is baking, combine the remaining ⅔ cup sugar, the cornstarch, and the remaining ¼ teaspoon salt in a heavy pan. Add the lemon juice and water to the pan and stir to combine. Bring the mixture to a gentle boil, stirring constantly, then boil for 1 minute, continuing to stir. Remove the pan from the heat, add the lemon zest, and let the contents cool completely.

When you're ready to assemble the shortcake, remove the peaches from the refrigerator and slice them. Whip the cream until it's stiff, then gently fold the whipped cream into the cooled cornstarch mixture. Transfer one cake layer, cut-side up, to a serving tray. Cover the layer with half the sliced peaches, then top the filling with half the lemon cream. Place the second layer on top, cut-side down, then cover it with the remaining peaches and cream.

Cut the shortcake into 10 sections to serve.

Nutritional Analysis

Per Serving

Calories (kcal)	459.5	Cholesterol (mg)	60.0
Total Fat (g)	14.5	Dietary Fiber (g)	2.4
Saturated Fat (g)	8.7	% Calories from Fat	27.9
Monounsaturated Fat (g)	4.2	Vitamin C (mg)	9.0
Polyunsaturated Fat (g)	0.7	Vitamin A (i.u.)	631.0

Gingerbread with Orange Sauce

If you have tasted only packaged gingerbread, this is a must—you'll never buy a box of gingerbread mix again!

Makes 8 servings

1 cup all-purpose flour

½ cup whole wheat flour

½ cup sugar

½ teaspoon baking soda

½ teaspoon baking powder

½ teaspoon plus ⅛ teaspoon salt

1 teaspoon ground cinnamon

½ teaspoon ground ginger

½ teaspoon ground allspice

½ teaspoon ground nutmeg

3 tablespoons butter, melted and cooled, plus 1 tablespoon butter

¼ cup pure maple syrup

½ cup low-fat (1%) milk

1 egg, well beaten

1½ tablespoons fresh orange juice

1 tablespoon cornstarch

¾ cup boiling water

½ teaspoon fresh lemon juice

Gingerbread

Preheat the oven to 350°F. Coat an 8-inch square baking pan with cooking spray.

Combine the flours, ¼ cup of the sugar, the baking soda, baking powder, the ½ teaspoon salt, and the spices in a large bowl. In a separate bowl mix the 3 tablespoons melted butter, the syrup, milk, and egg. Add the liquid to the dry ingredients and mix until the batter is smooth and creamy. Transfer the batter to the baking pan and bake the gingerbread for 25 minutes.

Orange Sauce

Mix the orange juice, the remaining ¼ cup sugar, the cornstarch, and the remaining ⅛ teaspoon salt in a saucepan. Place the pan over medium heat and add the boiling water. Bring the contents to a boil, reduce the heat, and simmer the sauce for 10 minutes, stirring occasionally. Add the lemon juice and the remaining 1 tablespoon butter and stir until the ingredients are well blended.

Serve the warm sauce on the gingerbread.

Nutritional Analysis

Per Serving

Calories (kcal)	228.5	Cholesterol (mg)	39.0
Total Fat (g)	6.8	Dietary Fiber (g)	1.6
Saturated Fat (g)	3.9	% Calories from Fat	26.2
Monounsaturated Fat (g)	1.9	Vitamin C (mg)	2.0
Polyunsaturated Fat (g)	0.4	Vitamin A (i.u.)	281.0

Hazelnut Meringue
with Raspberry Cream

*Egg whites make a terrific base for desserts without adding fat.
The wonderful toasty flavored hazelnuts add texture as well as a
great flavor. Without an egg- and butter-laden cake base, we can
even use a bit of whipped cream. Only 1 tablespoon of cream per
serving makes a tremendously rich dessert that is still low in fat!*

Makes 8 servings

¼ cup coarsely chopped
   hazelnuts

1¼ cups sugar

7 teaspoons cornstarch

8 egg whites, at room
   temperature

⅛ teaspoon salt

½ cup water

¼ cup pureed raspberries

½ cup whipping cream

Hazelnut Meringue

Preheat the oven to 350°F. Line a sheet pan (approximately 12" × 16"), or two
pans (approximately 6" × 8"), with parchment paper.

In a food processor, combine the hazelnuts, ⅔ cup of the sugar, and
4 teaspoons of the cornstarch and process the mixture until the nuts are finely
chopped.

Whip the egg whites until soft peaks form. Continue whipping and gradually
add ¼ cup of the remaining sugar, whipping until the meringue is very stiff.
Sprinkle one-third of the nut-sugar mixture over the meringue and gently fold
it in. Repeat with the remaining nut-sugar mixture, folding as gently as possible to keep the meringue fluffy. Spread the meringue evenly over the parchment paper and place the pan(s) in the oven. Immediately lower the heat to
250°F and bake the meringue for 3 hours, or until the tips are dry and crisp to
the touch. Loosen the edges with a knife and reverse the meringue onto a
rack. If one large pan has been used, cut the meringue in half into two 6" × 8"
rectangles. Carefully peel off the parchment. Let the meringue cool before
frosting.

Raspberry Cream

Combine the remaining ⅓ cup sugar, the remaining tablespoon of cornstarch, the salt, and water in a saucepan. Cook the mixture over medium heat, stirring constantly, until it becomes thick and clear. Boil the sauce gently for 1 minute. Remove the pan from the heat and allow the contents to cool.

When the sauce is cool, combine it well with the raspberries. Whip the cream until it's stiff and gently fold it into the raspberry mixture.

Place half of the raspberry cream on one layer of cooled meringue, top it with the second layer, and cover the top layer with the remaining cream. Serve the torte immediately or store it in the refrigerator until serving. This dessert may be made several hours ahead.

Nutritional Analysis

Per Serving

Calories (kcal)	212.7	Cholesterol (mg)	20.0
Total Fat (g)	6.8	Dietary Fiber (g)	0.4
Saturated Fat (g)	3.5	% Calories from Fat	28.2
Monounsaturated Fat (g)	2.6	Vitamin C (mg)	1.0
Polyunsaturated Fat (g)	0.3	Vitamin A (i.u.)	225.0

LEMON BARS

This treat tastes like bakery lemon bars, but the fat has been reduced to meet the guidelines for cancer risk reduction.

Makes 8 servings

1¼ cups all-purpose flour

1 cup whole wheat flour

1 cup granulated sugar

6 tablespoons butter, melted and cooled

1 teaspoon baking powder

3 eggs, beaten

6 tablespoons fresh lemon juice

1 teaspoon lemon zest

1 tablespoon sifted powdered sugar

Whole Wheat Crust

Preheat the oven to 350°F.

Mix 1 cup of the all-purpose flour, the whole wheat flour, and ½ cup of the granulated sugar; add the butter and mix the ingredients well. Press the dough onto the bottom of a 9" × 13" pan. Bake the crust for 20 minutes. Remove the pan from the oven, but leave the oven on. Set the baked crust aside and allow it to cool while you make the filling.

Lemon Filling

Mix the remaining ½ cup granulated sugar, the remaining ¼ cup flour, and the baking powder. Add the eggs, lemon juice, and lemon zest and mix well. Pour the lemon mixture over the cooled crust and bake for 25 minutes.

Sprinkle the powdered sugar over the top while the filling is still warm. Let the sheet cool slightly before cutting it into bars.

Nutritional Analysis

Per Serving

Calories (kcal)	323.9	Cholesterol (mg)	92.0
Total Fat (g)	10.6	Dietary Fiber (g)	2.5
Saturated Fat (g)	5.9	% Calories from Fat	28.7
Monounsaturated Fat (g)	3.1	Vitamin C (mg)	6.0
Polyunsaturated Fat (g)	0.7	Vitamin A (i.u.)	423.0

LEMON TART WITH MOSAIC OF FRUITS

Another version of a low-fat lemon tart, this dish is covered with a mosaic of bright oranges, peaches, and red raspberries. It only takes a short amount of time to make this dessert beautiful.

Makes 6 servings

3½ tablespoons butter, melted and cooled

¾ cup dry unseasoned bread crumbs

1 cup sugar

¼ cup cornstarch

1 cup water

2 egg yolks, beaten

3 tablespoons fresh lemon juice

1 tablespoon lemon zest

8 ounces fresh raspberries

1 peach, sliced thin

6 tablespoons raspberry jam

Preheat the oven to 400°F.

Mix 2 tablespoons of the butter with the bread crumbs and press the mixture onto the bottom a 10-inch tart or pie pan. Bake the crust for 10 minutes. Remove the pan from the oven, but leave the oven on. Cool the pan on a rack.

Combine the sugar and cornstarch in a saucepan. Whisk in the water. Bring the mixture to a boil and boil for about 20 seconds, stirring constantly, until the mixture is thickened. Remove the pan from the heat and allow the contents to cool a bit.

Pour some of the sugar mixture into the egg yolks, then return the mixture to the saucepan. Add the lemon juice, lemon zest, and the remaining 1½ tablespoons butter and stir to combine the ingredients. Pour the sauce into the shell and bake the tart for another 10 minutes. Allow the tart to cool, then top it with the raspberries and peach slices arranged in an attractive pattern. Heat the jam, let it cool a bit, and spoon it over the fruit.

Nutritional Analysis

Per Serving

Calories (kcal)	355.4	Cholesterol (mg)	89.0
Total Fat (g)	9.5	Dietary Fiber (g)	3.0
Saturated Fat (g)	4.9	% Calories from Fat	23.2
Monounsaturated Fat (g)	3.0	Vitamin C (mg)	16.0
Polyunsaturated Fat (g)	0.7	Vitamin A (i.u.)	467.0

PERSIMMON CAKE
WITH ORANGE-GINGER CREAM

*This is a favorite of our family and friends. The warm, dense cake
with the cool, light-textured cream is unbeatable!*

Makes 10 servings

3 tablespoons butter

1½ cups plus ⅔ cup sugar

2 tablespoons vanilla extract

2 eggs (keep separate)

2 pounds persimmons, peeled
and mashed

¼ cup milk

2¼ cups flour

1½ teaspoons baking soda

¾ teaspoon salt

1 teaspoon ground cinnamon

3 tablespoons orange zest

2 tablespoons cornstarch

⅓ cup fresh orange juice

1 cup water

1½ tablespoons candied minced
gingerroot

½ cup whipping cream

Persimmon Cake

Coat a 2-pound coffee can or pudding mold with cooking spray.

In a large bowl, combine the butter and the 1½ cups sugar with a fork until
the mixture is fluffy. Add the vanilla, then the eggs, one at a time, beating well
after each addition. Add the persimmon and milk, mixing well. Combine the
flour, soda, ½ teaspoon of the salt, the cinnamon, and 2 tablespoons of the
orange zest and add the dry ingredients to the persimmon mixture. Stir to
combine well.

Spoon the batter into the mold, cover it with foil, and tie the foil tightly with
string to keep water out.

Place the container on a rack or trivet in a deep pot. Add enough boiling
water to reach halfway up the container. Cover the pot and bring the water to
a boil; reduce the heat and let it simmer for 2 hours. Remove the container
from the pot and let the cake set for 10 minutes before unmolding it.

Orange-Ginger Cream

Combine the remaining ⅔ cup sugar, the cornstarch, and the remaining
¼ teaspoon salt in a heavy pan. Add the orange juice and water and stir to

combine. Bring the mixture to a gentle boil, stirring constantly until it is thickened. Boil 1 minute, stirring constantly. Remove the pan from the heat. Add the gingerroot and remaining tablespoon of orange zest. Let the contents cool completely.

Whip the cream until it's stiff and fold it into the cooled cornstarch mixture. The cream may be made several hours ahead and refrigerated.

Serve the cake warm with a dollop of orange-ginger cream.

Nutritional Analysis

Per Serving

Calories (kcal)	476.4	Cholesterol (mg)	64.0
Total Fat (g)	9.5	Dietary Fiber (g)	2.3
Saturated Fat (g)	5.3	% Calories from Fat	17.7
Monounsaturated Fat (g)	2.6	Vitamin C (mg)	56.0
Polyunsaturated Fat (g)	0.5	Vitamin A (i.u.)	375.0

POACHED WINTER FRUITS
WITH BLUEBERRY CAVIAR

*Despite its name, this dish could be made any time of the year—even
in the summer, using fresh blueberries. The colors are lovely,
and the slightly firm texture of the fruit, the soft caviar, and the crispy
macadamia nuts make a luscious dessert that contains
only 8.2 percent calories from fat.*

Makes 8 servings

4 apples, unpeeled

4 pears, unpeeled

2 cups water

1 cup fresh orange juice

1 cup plus 2 tablespoons sugar

1 teaspoon lemon zest

2 teaspoons vanilla extract

16 ounces frozen blueberries,
defrosted and undrained

2 tablespoons Grand Marnier
or orange juice

2 ounces macadamia nuts,
chopped coarse

Poached Fruit

Halve the apples and pears and remove the cores. Combine the water, orange
juice, the 1 cup sugar, the lemon zest, and 1 teaspoon of the vanilla in a large
pan and bring the mixture to a boil. Carefully add the apple, cut-side down,
reduce the heat to medium-low, and poach the apple for 5 minutes. Turn the
apple over and poach the fruit for 5 minutes longer. Lift the fruit out carefully and repeat the process with the pear, poaching the fruit for 5 minutes
per side.

The recipe may be made ahead up to this point (don't discard the poaching
liquid). At serving time, bring the poaching liquid to a simmer, carefully add
the apple and pear halves, and simmer the fruit just until they're warmed.

Blueberry Caviar

Puree the blueberries, the remaining 2 tablespoons sugar, the remaining
1 teaspoon vanilla, and the Grand Marnier until the mixture is almost smooth,
similar to the texture of caviar.

Place the poached fruit cut-side up on a platter. Fill each cavity with some of the blueberry caviar. Sprinkle the nuts on top just before serving.

Nutritional Analysis

Per Serving

Calories (kcal)	286.4	Cholesterol (mg)	0.2
Total Fat (g)	2.7	Dietary Fiber (g)	6.2
Saturated Fat (g)	1.4	% Calories from Fat	8.2
Monounsaturated Fat (g)	2.6	Vitamin C (mg)	25.0
Polyunsaturated Fat (g)	0.2	Vitamin A (i.u.)	108.0

Pumpkin Pie
with Oatmeal Cookie Crust

This is a low-fat alternative to traditional pumpkin pie. The oat crust adds interest, flavor, and texture as well as offering a lower-fat pie, since the crust has less butter than the usual shortening-laden piecrust.

Makes 10 servings

1 egg, slightly beaten, plus 2 whole eggs

3½ tablespoons butter, melted and cooled

2¼ cups rolled oats

6 tablespoons granulated sugar

1¾ teaspoons ground cinnamon

1 cup part-skim ricotta cheese

1 16-ounce can pumpkin

¾ cup brown sugar

½ teaspoon salt

1½ teaspoons pumpkin pie spice

1 teaspoon vanilla extract

1 5½-ounce can evaporated skim milk

¼ cup chopped walnuts

Oatmeal Crust

Preheat the oven to 350°F. Coat a 9" × 13" pan with cooking spray.

In a large bowl, combine the beaten egg with the butter. Add the oats, granulated sugar, and 1½ teaspoons of the cinnamon and combine the ingredients well. Press the mixture into the pan and bake the crust for 20 minutes. Remove the pan and raise the oven temperature to 375°F. Allow the crust to cool a bit before adding the filling.

Pumpkin Filling

Beat the remaining 2 eggs with the cheese, pumpkin, ½ cup of the brown sugar, the salt, pumpkin pie spice, vanilla, and evaporated milk until the mixture is well blended. Pour the filling into the cooled shell and bake the pie for 1 hour and 15 minutes.

Make the topping by combining the nuts, the remaining ¼ cup brown sugar, and the remaining ¼ teaspoon cinnamon. Sprinkle the nut topping over the pie directly after removing the pan from the oven. Allow the pie to cool a bit before serving.

Nutritional Analysis

Per Serving

Calories (kcal)	277.5	Cholesterol (mg)	74.0
Total Fat (g)	8.9	Dietary Fiber (g)	2.8
Saturated Fat (g)	4.3	% Calories from Fat	28.2
Monounsaturated Fat (g)	2.7	Vitamin C (mg)	3.0
Polyunsaturated Fat (g)	1.1	Vitamin A (i.u.)	929.0

Six-Layer Torte with Lemon Curd and Strawberries

*The beauty of this special "six-layer torte" is that the cake
may be purchased. You just make the lemon curd and layer it
with the strawberries in the cake. A lot of impact for little work!
And the fat content is very low for a torte of this type.*

Makes 8 servings

1 12-ounce angel food cake

1¼ cups plus ⅓ cup granulated
    sugar

1 tablespoon cornstarch

¼ teaspoon salt

¼ cup plus 3 tablespoons fresh
    lemon juice

½ cup water

½ teaspoon lemon zest

5 tablespoons butter

2 eggs plus 2 egg whites

12 ounces strawberries, washed
    and sliced

⅓ cup powdered sugar

Slice the cake horizontally into three layers.

In a heavy saucepan, combine the ⅓ cup granulated sugar, the cornstarch,
⅛ teaspoon salt, and the 3 tablespoons lemon juice with the water. Bring the
mixture slowly to a boil. Boil for 1 minute, whisking constantly. Remove the
pan from the heat, add the lemon zest, and set the pan aside to cool.

In another heavy pan, melt the butter. Add the remaining ¼ cup lemon juice,
the remaining ⅛ teaspoon salt, and the remaining 1¼ cups sugar, stirring until
the sugar is dissolved. In a bowl, beat the eggs and egg whites together until
they're well combined. Whisk some of the hot butter mixture into the eggs,
then add the entire egg mixture to the pan, whisking constantly. Cook the
contents gently, whisking constantly until the mixture is thick (about 15 minutes); do not allow it to boil. Remove the pan from the heat. Allow the mixture to cool, then combine it with the cooled cornstarch mixture.

Spread one-third of the lemon curd over the bottom cake layer and top it with one-third of the strawberries. Repeat the process with the second and third layers. Sprinkle the top layer with the powdered sugar.

Nutritional Analysis

Per Serving

Calories (kcal)	383.4	Cholesterol (mg)	65.0
Total Fat (g)	8.4	Dietary Fiber (g)	1.0
Saturated Fat (g)	4.8	% Calories from Fat	19.2
Monounsaturated Fat (g)	2.5	Vitamin C (mg)	29.0
Polyunsaturated Fat (g)	0.5	Vitamin A (i.u.)	346.0

Spicy Pumpkin Pie

This flavorful pumpkin pie leaves no room for complaints that "pumpkin pie is too bland." It has loads of flavor, and keeping the filling low in fat allows for the use of a traditional piecrust (which is much too high in fat to use with a high-fat filling).

Makes 8 servings

1 9-inch piecrust (homemade, or purchased ready-made)

1 egg white plus 2 eggs, slightly beaten, plus 2 additional egg whites

½ cup sugar

3 tablespoons molasses

1 teaspoon salt

1 tablespoon ground cinnamon

1 tablespoon ground ginger

1 teaspoon ground allspice

1 teaspoon ground nutmeg

2½ cups canned pumpkin puree

1 cup low-fat (1%) milk

Preheat the oven to 450°F.

Lightly brush the pie shell with the beaten egg white. Whisk the 2 beaten eggs with the sugar, molasses, salt, and spices until the ingredients are well combined. Stir in the pumpkin and milk, mixing well. Stiffly beat the 2 remaining egg whites and fold them into the pumpkin mixture. Pour the filling into the crust, mounding the filling in center.

Bake the pie at 450°F for 15 minutes; lower the temperature to 375°F and bake for 15 minutes longer; then reduce the temperature to 350°F and bake for 45 more minutes, or until a knife inserted in the center comes out clean.

Nutritional Analysis

Per Serving

Calories (kcal)	236.7	Cholesterol (mg)	47.0
Total Fat (g)	7.9	Dietary Fiber (g)	3.2
Saturated Fat (g)	2.3	% Calories from Fat	29.1
Monounsaturated Fat (g)	4.0	Vitamin C (mg)	4.0
Polyunsaturated Fat (g)	0.9	Vitamin A (i.u.)	7,021.0

Sugar Cookies

This is the only recipe in the book that requires margarine instead of butter. Egg whites are used instead of whole eggs; extra flour helps make up for the change in consistency of the dough because of the reduction in fat.

Makes 6 dozen cookies; 1 cookie per serving

1 cup soft tub margarine (no substitutions)

2 cups sugar

4 egg whites (keep separate)

¼ cup skim milk

1 tablespoon vanilla extract

5½ cups flour

1 tablespoon baking powder

½ teaspoon salt

Beat the margarine with the sugar until the mixture is fluffy. Beat in the egg whites (one at a time), milk, and vanilla and mix well. Combine the flour, baking powder, and salt, and blend the dry ingredients into the margarine mixture.

On a floured board, shape the dough into two 12" × 2½" logs. Wrap the logs well in plastic wrap and refrigerate them for 1 hour (or freeze until needed*).

Preheat the oven to 375°F.

Slice each roll into 36 cookies and decorate them, if desired. Transfer the cookies to an ungreased baking sheet (lined with parchment paper for easy cleanup), and bake for 10 to 12 minutes. Dot the warm cookies with colored sprinkles or tiny silver candies (sold in the baking goods section of a supermarket).

Variation

This dough can be put through a cookie press to make spritz or other pressed cookies.

---

*If the dough is to be frozen, wrap the logs in plastic wrap, then overwrap them in foil or place them in a freezer zip-style bag. Defrost the logs at room temperature before cutting.

Nutritional Analysis

Per Serving

Calories (kcal)	80.8	Cholesterol (mg)	0.0
Total Fat (g)	2.6	Dietary Fiber (g)	0.3
Saturated Fat (g)	0.4	% Calories from Fat	29.2
Monounsaturated Fat (g)	1.0	Vitamin C (mg)	0.0
Polyunsaturated Fat (g)	1.0	Vitamin A (i.u.)	106.0

Three-Citrus Meringue Tart

Don't be alarmed by the length of this recipe—it's not complicated, but the depth of flavor from the combination of citrus fruits is well worth the moderate amount of time it takes to make. It can be prepared one day ahead, except for the final step of making the meringue.

Makes 6 servings

½ cup plus 1½ tablespoons flour

½ cup sugar

2 tablespoons butter, melted

½ teaspoon baking powder

¼ teaspoon salt

5 egg whites (keep separate) plus 1 whole egg

2 tablespoons fresh lemon juice

2 tablespoons fresh orange juice

2 tablespoons fresh lime juice

1 teaspoon lemon zest

1 teaspoon orange zest

1 teaspoon lime zest

⅛ teaspoon cream of tartar

Tart Crust

Preheat the oven to 350°F. Coat an 8-inch square baking pan with cooking spray.

Combine the ½ cup flour and 2 tablespoons of the sugar in a large bowl. Add the butter and stir the mixture with a fork until coarse crumbs form (the mixture will be dry). With your fingers, press the crumbs over the bottom of the baking pan. Bake the crust until it is set and light golden, about 20 minutes. Remove the pan, but leave the oven on. Allow the crust to cool completely on a rack.

Citrus Filling

Mix ¼ cup of the remaining sugar, the remaining 1½ tablespoons flour, the baking powder, and salt in a small bowl. Whisk 3 of the egg whites, the whole egg, the juices, and ¾ teaspoon each of the zests in a medium bowl. Add the flour mixture and whisk until the sauce is smooth. Pour the filling over the cooled crust. Bake the tart until the filling is set, about 18 minutes. Remove the pan from the oven, but if you are going to make the meringue next, leave the oven on. Allow the tart to cool completely on a rack. (The filled tart can be made 1 day ahead. Cover and refrigerate.)

Meringue

Beat the remaining 2 egg whites and the cream of tartar in a large, clean bowl until soft peaks form. Add the remaining 2 tablespoons sugar, 1 tablespoon at a time, and beat until stiff peaks form. Spoon the meringue over the filling, covering it completely. Sprinkle the remaining ¼ teaspoon each of the zests on top. Bake the meringue until the tips begin to brown, about 10 minutes.

Transfer the pan to a rack. Allow the tart to cool completely before cutting.

Nutritional Analysis

Per Serving

Calories (kcal)	172.8	Cholesterol (mg)	40.0
Total Fat (g)	4.6	Dietary Fiber (g)	0.5
Saturated Fat (g)	2.6	% Calories from Fat	23.8
Monounsaturated Fat (g)	1.4	Vitamin C (mg)	8.0
Polyunsaturated Fat (g)	0.3	Vitamin A (i.u.)	191.0

21-Day Menu Plan II

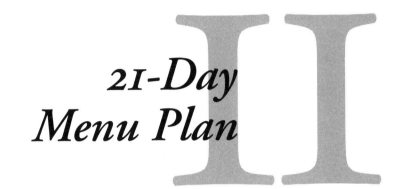

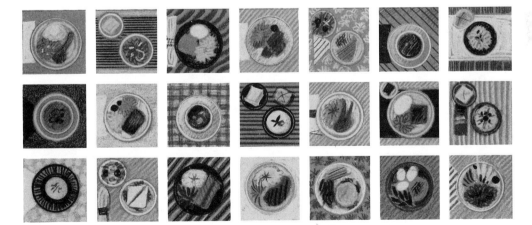

An asterisk (*) indicates that the recipe is in the book (see Index). Menus are based on approximately 1,800 calories per day.

DAY 1: 1,848.50 CALORIES—47.52 GRAMS FIBER

Breakfast

1 cup fresh blackberries
2 Oat Bran Muffins*
1 cup low-fat (1%) milk

Lunch

1 bowl split pea soup
Spinach salad (2 cups spinach, 1 sliced carrot, and 1½ tablespoons vinaigrette)
1 slice pumpernickel bread

Dinner

Peppercorn Steaks with Noodles and Cabernet Sauce*
½ cup broccoli
1 orange

DAY 2: 1,603.30 CALORIES—36.35 GRAMS FIBER

Breakfast

1 cup strawberry yogurt with ½ cup sliced strawberries and ¼ cup Fiber One cereal
1 slice whole wheat bread

Lunch

Turkey sandwich (2 slices whole wheat bread, 4 ounces turkey, 1 medium sliced tomato, ½ cup romaine, and 1 tablespoon mayonnaise)
1 carrot
1 apple

Dinner

Linguine with Clam Sauce*

1 cup asparagus with 1½ tablespoons vinaigrette

Fruit cup (1 banana, ½ cup seedless grapes, and 1 orange)

DAY 3: 1,632.57 CALORIES—39.44 GRAMS FIBER

Breakfast

1 cup oatmeal with 1 sliced banana, ⅓ cup raisins, and 2 tablespoons pure
   maple syrup

6 ounces fresh orange juice

Lunch

Tuna salad (2 cups romaine, 4 ounces tuna in water, ½ cup chopped green bell
   pepper, ½ cup chopped celery, ¼ cup chopped scallion, and 2 tablespoons
   ranch dressing)

1 cup fresh pineapple

Dinner

Onion-Fried Mandarin Orange Chicken* served over 1 cup brown rice

½ cup peas with 2 teaspoons mint jelly

DAY 4: 1,571.90 CALORIES—38.29 GRAMS FIBER

Breakfast

Oatmeal Breakfast Bread*

½ cup raspberries

1 cup low-fat (1%) milk

Lunch

1 bowl minestrone soup

2 slices French bread with 2 ounces part-skim mozzarella cheese

1 peach

Dinner

Mexican Chicken with Salsa and Rice*

½ cup corn

1 cup raspberries with ¼ cup vanilla ice milk

DAY 5: 1,721.20 CALORIES—50.62 GRAMS FIBER

Breakfast

Mushroom omelet (1 egg, 2 egg whites, ¼ cup sliced mushrooms, and
2 tablespoons chopped scallion cooked in a nonstick pan with 1 teaspoon
butter)

2 slices rye bread

1½ cups cubed cantaloupe

Lunch

4 ounces canned salmon on 2 slices whole wheat bread with ½ tablespoon
mayonnaise and 1 cucumber, sliced thin

2 apricots

Dinner

Turkey Scaloppine with Lemon Cream Sauce*

1 baked potato (spoon some of the scaloppine sauce on top)

6 ounces artichoke hearts served with 1½ tablespoons Hoisin-Orange
Vinaigrette*

1 slice peach pie (bakery style)

Day 6: 1,757.00 Calories—42.50 Grams Fiber

Breakfast

1 oatmeal bagel

2 tablespoons low-fat cream cheese

1 cup blackberries with 2 tablespoons blackberry yogurt

Lunch

Roast beef sandwich (3 ounces roast beef, ½ tomato, ½ cup sprouts, ¼ green bell pepper, and 1 tablespoon mayonnaise on a whole wheat English muffin)

1½ cups sliced papaya

Dinner

Chili-Cheese Pie*

Crudités—1 sliced carrot, 1 sliced red bell pepper, and 1 cup broccoli florets, with 3 tablespoons blue cheese dressing as dip (low-fat variety found in supermarket refrigerated section)

2 oatmeal cookies

Day 7: 1,711.70 Calories—39.36 Grams Fiber

Breakfast

½ cup Bran Buds with ½ cup low-fat (1%) milk, 1 sliced banana, and ¼ cup raisins

6 ounces fresh orange juice

Lunch

Chicken Caesar salad (3 cups romaine, 4 ounces boneless, skinless chicken breast, and 2 tablespoons Caesar salad dressing)

1 piece Corn Bread*

Dinner

Shrimp Jambalaya*

½ cup steamed broccoli with 1½ tablespoons vinaigrette

1 sweet potato with ½ tablespoon butter

DAY 8: 1,799.40 CALORIES—35.67 GRAMS FIBER

Breakfast

Apple-Cranberry Cobbler*

1 cup low-fat (1%) milk

1 pear

Lunch

1 10-ounce beef-and-bean burrito

¾ cup Spanish-style rice

1 apple

Dinner

1½ cups Manhattan clam chowder

Shrimp salad (3 cups romaine, 6 ounces shrimp, 3 ounces artichoke hearts, and 2 tablespoons Thousand Island dressing)

½ grapefruit with 1 tablespoon brown sugar, broiled

DAY 9: 1,866.50 CALORIES—33.66 GRAMS FIBER

Breakfast

1 cup oatmeal with ½ cup sliced strawberries and 1 tablespoon maple syrup

1 cup low-fat (1%) milk

Lunch

Grilled chicken sandwich (2 slices pumpernickel bread, 4 ounces boneless, skinless chicken breast, and 2 tablespoons reduced-fat Thousand Island dressing)

2 cups mixed fruit

Dinner

Thyme-Crusted Pork Tenderloin*

Steamed broccoli and cauliflower florets (¾ cup each) with 1½ tablespoons butter

1 cup blackberries with ½ cup blackberry ice cream

DAY 10: 1,858.70 CALORIES—34.94 GRAMS FIBER

Breakfast

1 slice whole wheat bread with 1 tablespoon peanut butter

1 banana

1 cup low-fat (1%) milk

Lunch

Spinach-Cheese Pancakes*

Braised Fresh Tomatoes*

2 cups cubed watermelon

Dinner

Asian beef salad (4 ounces lean sandwich-style beef [from the deli] cut in strips, tossed with 2 cups bean sprouts, 1 cup sugar snap peas, ¼ cup chopped scallion, ¼ cup chopped fresh cilantro, 1 tablespoon salad dressing—preferably Asian-style, and 1 tablespoon soy sauce)

1 orange, peeled and sliced

2 fortune cookies

Day 11: 1,795.95 calories—34.67 grams fiber

Breakfast

Fried egg sandwich (2 slices cracked wheat toast, with 1 egg fried in a nonstick skillet and condiments of choice)

1 cup unsweetened applesauce

Lunch

Crab melt (4 ounces crab mixed with ¼ cup celery, 2 tablespoons scallion, and 1 tablespoon mayonnaise—spread on a split whole wheat English muffin, sprinkled with ¼ cup grated part-skim mozzarella cheese, then broiled)

6 ounces V-8 juice

1 peach

Dinner

4 ounces roasted chicken (from the deli)

Mustard-Cream Broccoli and Carrots*

2 whole wheat dinner rolls with ½ tablespoon butter

1 serving Ambrosia*

Day 12: 1,814.30 calories—34.53 grams fiber

Breakfast

2 slices pumpernickel toast spread with 2 tablespoons low-fat cream cheese, sprinkled with chives

1½ cups sliced mango or cantaloupe

Lunch

Stouffer's Chinese Green Pepper Steak (with rice)

Carrots in Fresh Basil Vinaigrette*

1 orange

6 ounces V-8 juice

Dinner

Oven-Roasted Lamb with Vegetable Sauce*

¾ cup sliced, steamed carrots

1 cup raspberries with ½ cup raspberry ice cream and ½ cup granola

DAY 13: 1,403.00 CALORIES—39.43 GRAMS FIBER

Breakfast

½ cup Fiber One cereal with 4 ounces low-fat (1%) milk and 1 sliced peach

1 slice cracked wheat toast with ½ tablespoon butter

Lunch

Stouffer's Spaghetti with Beef and Mushroom Sauce (Lean Cuisine)

Salad (2 cups romaine, 1 grated carrot, and 1½ tablespoons vinaigrette)

Dinner

4 ounces roast turkey breast (homemade or deli)

Chardonnay Applesauce with Sweet Onion and Thyme*

1½ cups steamed broccoli florets with fresh lemon juice

1 cup winter squash with ½ tablespoon butter

2 oatmeal cookies

1 cup low-fat (1%) milk

DAY 14: 1,629.35 CALORIES—37.82 GRAMS FIBER

Breakfast

1 cup mixed berries (½ cup each blueberries and raspberries)

1 cup nonfat milk

2 Corn Muffins*

Lunch

1 6-ounce Weight Watcher's Cheese Pizza

Crudités—1 sliced carrot, 1 sliced celery stalk, and ½ sliced green bell pepper with 2 tablespoons (light) blue cheese dressing as dip

1½ cups cubed cantaloupe

Dinner

4 ounces lean roasted pork tenderloin (homemade or deli)

Cranberry Salsa*

¾ cup peas with 1 tablespoon mint jelly

Vermicelli-Rice Pilaf*

Day 15: 1,833.70 calories—52.10 grams fiber

Breakfast

1 cup vanilla yogurt with 1 sliced peach, sprinkled with ¼ cup Fiber One cereal

1 blueberry muffin

Lunch

Black Bean Soup with Tomatillos*

2 corn tortillas

1 cup fresh pineapple

Dinner

Provençale chicken sandwich (1 French roll, 4 ounces grilled chicken breast, ¼ cup roasted red peppers, 2 tablespoons feta, and 3 olives)

2 chopped tomatoes with 2 tablespoons chopped fresh basil and 1 tablespoon olive oil

3 quartered figs drizzled with 2 tablespoons warm honey

Day 16: 1,526.4 Calories—32.75 Grams Fiber

Breakfast
Vanilla-Walnut Granola* with 1 cup low-fat (1%) milk and ½ cup blackberries

1 whole wheat English muffin

Lunch
1 bowl tomato soup with ½ cup brown rice and ¼ cup cheddar cheese
   sprinkled on top

3 slices white meat chicken on a bed of Chinese cabbage or mixed greens

Drizzle with low-fat, low-calorie salad dressing

Dinner
4 ounces grilled salmon fillet

2 cups steamed Swiss chard

2 ounces (dry) linguini, cooked, and tossed with 1 tablespoon olive oil
   and 1 or 2 cloves minced garlic

1½ cups cantaloupe balls, with ½ cup blueberries and 2 tablespoons low-fat
   blueberry yogurt

Day 17: 1,923.50 Calories—43.17 Grams Fiber

Breakfast
Norwegian Pancakes* with 2 tablespoons maple syrup

1 cup sliced strawberries

1 cup fresh orange juice

Lunch
Mixed green salad (2 cups romaine, ¼ cup chopped onion, ½ cup each
   chopped celery and cucumber, and 2 tablespoons vinaigrette)

3 ounces shrimp

1 tangerine

Dinner

Hummus*

1 falafel

1 whole wheat pita round

1 cup broccoli florets tossed with 1 tablespoon olive oil and ½ teaspoon minced garlic

2 apricots

Day 18: 1,716.60 calories—40.11 grams fiber

Breakfast

1 bagel with 2 tablespoons low-fat cream cheese

2 ounces turkey pastrami or turkey ham

8 ounces orange juice

Lunch

White Bean–Tomatillo Chili with Cilantro-Cream Salsa*

¼ cup shredded cheddar cheese (for topping, if desired)

8 baked tortilla chips (2 corn tortillas cut in triangles and baked)

1 cup sliced strawberries

Dinner

4 ounces flank steak

1 cup steamed carrots

1 cup asparagus tips

1 medium baked potato with 2 tablespoons low-fat sour cream

Day 19: 1,700.39 calories—42.24 grams fiber

Breakfast

Breakfast shake (1 cup fresh orange juice, 1 cup low-fat strawberry yogurt, and ½ cup strawberries pureed in a blender)

1 whole wheat English muffin with 2 tablespoons jam

Lunch

2 cups fresh spinach tossed with 4 ounces shrimp and 1½ tablespoons vinaigrette

1 piece Corn Bread*, split and toasted, spread with ½ tablespoon butter

1 apple

Dinner

4 ounces roasted chicken breast (homemade or deli)

Roasted Balsamic Onions*

1 baked sweet potato, split, with 2 tablespoons fresh orange juice

2 cups mixed greens (dark, such as mustard), 1 sliced cucumber, and 2 tablespoons (light) blue cheese dressing

DAY 20: 1,523.50 CALORIES—37.38 GRAMS FIBER

Breakfast

2 Oat Bran Muffins*

Fruit cup (1 banana, 1 orange, and ½ cup sliced strawberries)

Lunch

Tuna sandwich (2 slices cracked wheat bread, 3 ounces tuna in water, 1½ tablespoons mayonnaise, 1 tomato, and ½ cup chopped romaine)

2 carrots, cut into sticks

1 tangerine

Dinner

3 ounces cold sliced (or cubed) lean beef

2 cups steamed greens (such as kale or mustard), tossed with 1 tablespoon olive oil and ½ teaspoon minced garlic

½ cup brown rice with ½ tablespoon butter

Blackberry Cantaloupe*

Day 21: 1,917 calories—38.7 grams fiber

Breakfast

1 cup oatmeal with ¼ cup pureed raspberries

1 whole wheat English muffin with ½ tablespoon butter

1 cup orange juice

Lunch

Quick pizza (1 whole wheat pita round, 2 tablespoons tomato sauce, 2 ounces grated cheddar cheese, and ¼ cup sliced mushrooms—broiled)

Salad (2 cups romaine, 1 grated carrot, and 1½ tablespoons vinaigrette)

1 orange

Dinner

Spicy Thai Tofu*

Asian broccoli (2 cups broccoli florets tossed with 1 tablespoon each canola oil and low-sodium soy sauce)

Frozen yogurt parfait (1 cup frozen nonfat yogurt and 1 cup blackberries—alternate 3 layers of each)

APPENDIX

Complete Protein Combinations

You will be eating a "complete protein" when you consume foods in the combinations shown. Where the circles overlap, you have a complete protein if there is a plus (+) sign. In the overlap area with a minus (–) sign, you need to add a food from the legume group to make a complete protein.

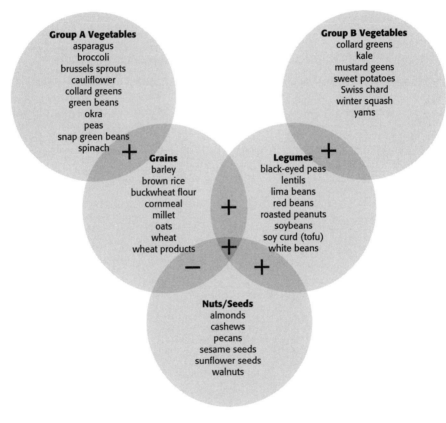

Group A Vegetables
asparagus
broccoli
brussels sprouts
cauliflower
collard greens
green beans
okra
peas
snap green beans
spinach

Group B Vegetables
collard greens
kale
mustard geens
sweet potatoes
Swiss chard
winter squash
yams

Grains
barley
brown rice
buckwheat flour
cornmeal
millet
oats
wheat
wheat products

Legumes
black-eyed peas
lentils
lima beans
red beans
roasted peanuts
soybeans
soy curd (tofu)
white beans

Nuts/Seeds
almonds
cashews
pecans
sesame seeds
sunflower seeds
walnuts

Examples

- Combine beans, peas, or lentils with rice
- Combine broccoli or cauliflower with whole wheat pasta
- Combine winter squash with lentil soup
- Sprinkle sunflower seeds on a salad with kidney beans
- Spread peanut butter on whole-grain bread

INDEX